The Home Health Aide Textbook

Home Care Principles

2nd Edition

Jane John-Nwankwo RN, MSN

THE HOME HEALTH AIDE TEXTBOOK: Home Care Principles

2nd Edition.

Copyright © 2015 by Jane John-Nwankwo RN, MSN

www.janejohn-nwankwo.com

ISBN-13: 978-1511736329

ISBN-10: 1511736321

Printed in the United States of America

Dedication

To my love, John Nwankwo Sr. and my sweet disciples:

Jessica, John Jr. and Joy.

Table of Contents

Introduction

This book was written out of an inner passion to provide a quality, but concise textbook for Home Health Aides as well as Caregivers. If the reader gains any new knowledge from this book or finds new strength to care for people who require care in their homes, then the purpose of this book would have been achieved.

- Jane John-Nwankwo RN, MSN.

Chapter One

Introduction to the Home Health Agency Role

Outline

1. Introduction

2. State and federal regulations and requirements for HHA certification

3. Purpose and goals of home health care

4. Members of the home health care team

5. Roles and responsibilities of the certified home health aide

6. Common observations and documentation to be done by the HHA

7. Key steps in the communication process and methods of communication

8. Key steps in accommodating communication with clients with hearing or speech disorders.

9. Effective techniques for communication with home health team members

10. Effective communication in learning about clients.

11. Access to community agencies to meet client needs

12. Organizational and time management techniques for a daily work schedule.

13. Conclusion

I. State and Federal Regulations and the requirements for HHA Certification

According to Davila (n.d.), to become a home health aide, there is no standardized national educational requirement. It depends on which state the HHA is in. While in some states, they don't need any state approved training, other states need them to take state approved classes, pass a competency test and earn a state certification. These classes are usually offered in the community colleges or vocational/technical schools.

Most skill training for HHAs are taught by other healthcare professionals like nurses, and is usually administered during the training period. Usually their training is moduled around the unique needs of home care clients. They also receive orientation on the job. Depending on the level of care needed by the client, the HHA's training could be done from a few hours to a few days. For more complex cases, some employers provide training classes which the aspiring HHA has to pass before they are given a job. Most employers would rather hire a Certified Home Health Aide, than an uncertified caregiver. The HHA certification process includes at least 75 hours of training and as much as a 120 hour course in a state like California. It involves the theory section of the training and the skills section. Other requirements may include a background check of candidates before enrolling them to a program due to the high trust nature of the job. Sometimes, physical examinations and health screenings like a tuberculosis test may be required to prevent patients from contracting diseases from their caregivers.

II. Purpose and goals of Home Health Care

Home Health Care involves a range of care for a wide variety of patients outside the hospital setting. The services that home health care companies provide can range from nursing care, physical therapy, occupational therapy, speech therapy, etc. from qualified medical professionals to smaller services from home health aides. The care provided could be as simple as assistance in everyday activities such as bathing and eating, to more complex services requiring more specialized professionals. Essentially, the purpose and goal of home care is to provide an adequate level of care in a cost-effective manner while promoting rehabilitation of the patient in a familiar environment like their homes.

III. Members of the home health care team

Physician - Physicians perform home visits to the patient at regular intervals where they assess the patient in an environment that the patient is more comfortable in. They assess how the patient handles his illness at home. The physician regularly checks and makes adjustments and interventions when necessary. There are two ways in which a physician can function in the Home health care setting. One of them relies on the home health care nurse as the leader, mediator, and coordinator of the group, leaving the physician to be an evaluator of the patient's health to be coordinated with the rest of the team by the nurse. The other way that the physician can function is to be the one who will lead the team by taking a more active role in patient care. The physician writes prescriptions for the home care client. At the patient's home, the nurses will be able to get a more in-depth assessment of the aspects of the patient's life that is not normally accessible from the hospital setting. In the home, the nurse can look for environmental factors found in the home that could affect the patient's illness, they could see how the patient acts in a more comfortable setting than a hospital, they can assess the patient's compliance with the therapeutic regimen, including diet, exercise, and medications. From these observations, the Registered Nurse can identify some areas that need adjustment in the patient's activities and make interventions to change them for the patient's health. They can also assess the tasks of the health care team and change them to better suit the therapeutic regimen, especially if the Registered Nurse is the one functioning as team leader and coordinator.

Nurse - Most of the care in Home health care is rendered by the nurse. The nurse collaborates with the physician to give the patient the proper care that he needs. They also work with the rest of the personnel in the home health care team to coordinate the services being provided to make sure the patient gets optimal service from each of them to improve the patient's quality of life at home. They perform different nursing interventions adjusted in frequency to suit the patient's needs. During the initial assessment, they also decide which of the other ancillary services are needed by the patient, and this is relayed to the physician who makes the final decision. The nurse's recommendations influence the interventions ordered by the physician. The treatment plans change based on the changes noted by the nurse since they spend the most time with the patient. Because of this, they are the ones in the position to make the comprehensive problems lists and the assessment of care and goal plans. When there are multiple therapies to be done by different members of the home health care team, the nurse schedules the interventions in a way in which they do not overlap so as not to inconvenience the team or stress the patient. Perhaps one of the most important responsibilities of the nurse is the documentation. They compile all the data about the patient including the treatment plans, prescriptions, and assessments. This serves as a valuable resource to be used by the whole health care team, and serves as proof that the team is doing their job. Nurses are also the ones who stay in contact with the whole team, and other community services that could be involved in the patient's care. The nurse updates the rest of the team and allows sharing of information through case conferences.

Pharmacist - The role of the pharmacist in the home health care setting is to be responsible for the patient's or caregiver's willingness and ability to be trained to properly administer medications, including the appropriate indications, dose, route, method of administration, and appropriate laboratory tests to monitor the patient's response to the pharmacologic therapy. They use their clinical judgement as to whether the first dose of any drug should be given at the home. It is their job to teach the caregiver about the medications, their effects, adverse effects, any drug interactions, storage and preparation, disposal, special precautions, and general management of drug effects, including emergency procedures. They also make sure that the patient does not run out of medications by checking their stock and by directing them to where they could get medical supplies. The pharmacist works together with the other health care professionals, the patient, and the caregiver in ensuring the appropriate pharmaceutical treatment plan for the patient. They must always be available in case there are any problems, questions, or concerns regarding the pharmacologic treatments. It is important for home health aides to check their state regulations before assisting with medications because most states do not allow HHAs to administer medications.

Physical therapist - The physical therapist is needed when the patient has trouble ambulating or has a disability that prevents him from performing everyday tasks. It is their job to assess the patient's disability to determine if the patient needs assistive devices. Once a patient is eligible for an assistive device, the physical therapist has to be the one to teach the patient its proper use. He also helps the patient increase his mobility and reduce risks of injuries from accidents. He creates the home exercise program to help the patient move around more. During every visit, he assesses the patient's mobility and adjusts the exercises as appropriate to the patient's range of motion, muscle strength, and endurance.

Occupational therapist - The occupational therapist is concerned with how the patient's disease or disability affects their ability to function normally. It is their job to help patients achieve a higher level of independence in everyday tasks such as bathing, dressing, elimination, cooking, eating, and housework. They provide the patient with information about various techniques, equipment, and aids that would allow them to function through their disability. They can help the patient make adjustments to their homes and belongings to improve the patient's functionality; they can teach energy conservation techniques for patients who have low endurance; they are also the ones to teach patients to use specially designed devices to increase their autonomy and functionality. By allowing the patient to do more by himself or herself, their self-esteem increases, and can decrease the need for constant supervision.

These therapists manipulate the environment of the patient to make it easier for the patient to function, such as widening doors for wheelchairs, grab rails, guide rails, placing objects and switches within arm's reach of the patient, adjusting furniture for easier travel around the house, etc.

Speech therapist - The speech therapist helps patients recover and develop their communication skills for those who have lost the ability to speak normally. They teach compensatory communication mechanisms that uses visual cues and cognitive retraining. They use a wide range of communication aids and technology such as hearing aids, or an electrolarynx; they also teach sign language, and the use of communication boards. As technology for the speech impaired increases, some speech therapist can even teach patients in the usage of transcription technology which transcribes spoken words onto a computer screen.

Social worker - The social worker provides emotional and psychological support to the home care team. The social worker is the one with access to community care services when there are conflicts with the treatment plant or if the patient refuses care. When more support is needed in the care of the patient, the social worker assesses the patient with regards to mobility, personal care ability, including an assessment of finances if the patient could afford another professional on the team. They also include the assessments of the rest of the home care team in the making of this decision. The social worker is the link to formal and informal sources of support, whether it comes from social groups, organizations, or help groups. The social worker coordinates, teaches, counsels, assesses, and facilitates ethical decision making issues. They also maintain standards by regular visits and inspections. They are available through a 24 hour emergency call system for the elderly and disabled.

Home Health Aide - The home health aide fulfills the personal care role for the patient. They do the daily tasks of bathing, clothing, positioning, and environmental care of the patient under the supervision of the home care nurse (Kurashi, 2006).

IV. Roles and responsibilities of the certified home health aide.

The certified home health aides fulfill the personal care role for the patient. These healthcare professionals perform under the guidance of the home care nurse, following a written care plan outlining activities and tasks to be done for the patient. This includes the basic tasks of bathing the patient, helping the patient sit upright, position, off, and on to bed, grooming, dental hygiene, basic exercises, and medication. Sometimes, HHAs may help in some household chores such as changing bed linens and keeping the patient's room clean as part of environmental care. Some of these jobs can be done by a trained paid housekeeper. Family members are also candidates for the role of a home health aide (Kurashi, 2006) if they undergo proper training.

V. Common observations and documentation to be done by the HHA.

According to the Home Health Aide Training Manual by
Kay Green (1996), the frequent observations of the HHA
include general observations such as weight changes,
changes in ability to perform care, ingestion of alcohol or
drugs, fevers, or episodes of weakness; skin observations
such as rashes, breaks or tears, changes in color, itching, or
bruises; head observations such as headaches, dizziness,
fainting spells, and hallucinations; eye observations such as
failing eyesight, excessive watering of the eyes, or dryness
of the eyes; Ear observations including hearing ability,
tinnitus, or discharge from the ears; nose and throat
observations including congestion, voice changes,
nosebleeds, toothaches, patient's dental hygiene, bleeding
gums, difficulty swallowing, and halitosis; breast
observations such as nipple discharges, lumps, or pains;
respiratory system observations including shortness of
breath, abnormal breath sounds, coughing, or fluid filled
lungs; heart or vascular system observations involving the
patient's heart rate, the regularity of his heartbeat, and any
chest pains; Stomach and intestinal observations such as the
patient's appetite, abdominal discomfort, diarrhea,
constipation, vomiting, blood in the stools, and
incontinence; urinary system observations such as the
patient's frequency of urination, the color of the urine,

incontinence, blood in the urine, the amount of urine, and any pain or difficulty in urination; observations of the patient's genitals such as any abnormal discharges, pain, lesions, and other abnormalities; observations of the patient's musculature such as muscle weakness, neck or back pain, joint pain, cramps, and limitations to movement; Changes in mental/emotional state such as crying, depression, nervousness, and restlessness; and finally neurological system observations such as seizures, numbness, tingling, paralysis, or loss of function. All these observations are to be documented along with the activities done by the HHA during his shift.

All these are documented for the benefit of the patient, the home health care team, and the HHA himself. By documenting these details, the patient's condition can be tracked, and the health care team can identify incremental changes in his condition to adjust the care plan accordingly, while it also protects the HHA since the documentation is a reflection that the HHA is doing his job correctly.

VI. Key steps in the communication process and methods of communication

The key steps in the communication process are Creation, Transmission, Reception, Translation, and Response.

Methods of communication, especially in the home health care setting consist of verbal and non-verbal modes of communication such as written communication (Schreiner, n.d.). Since the HHA has the most contact with the home care client, it is imperative that he reports any changes in the patient condition that is noticed. He should ensure that the data is being transmitted to the right personnel to avoid a breach of patient confidentiality. Clarity in communication is also very essential, avoiding the use of unnecessary abbreviations. E.g. The PT visited the PT. This could mean that the Physical therapist visited the patient, it could also mean that the patient went to the physical therapist office. In any case, there could arise some confusion as to the actual meaning of the documentation. Write in clear simple language that everyone can understand. Avoid cancellations, and if there be a need for cancellations, use only one line across your documentation.

VII. Key steps in accommodating communication with clients with hearing or speech disorders.

It is prudent to keep in mind that this type of communication is difficult, so patience is needed. The nurse must speak in short, clear sentences; do not use a lot of jargon; use communication tools such as pen and paper, pictures, or sign language if the patient has been taught; If the patient cannot speak, ask yes or no questions instead; use communication aids; consult a speech therapist ("Communicating with patients who have speech/language difficulties," 2009). The HHA must speak in a clear manner, loud enough for the patient to hear but at the same time, not shouting. If the client hears better with one hear, stand closer to the ear with a better function. Facing the client with hearing difficulty is often helpful since most of them compensate with lip reading. Never be in a hurry when communicating with clients with hearing or speech disorder; allow them time to finish their sentences and do not assume that you know what they have in mind to say. Encouraging sign language when the client is being trained to recover their speech abilities is not a good rehabilitation technique.

VIII. Effective techniques for communication with home health team members

One of the most effective techniques for communication, and the most important, is the written form of communication of the documentation. This record of everything done by, to, and about the patient is meant to be a non-urgent form of communication between the health team members. It should be regularly updated so that the other team members will be abreast of the patient's current status, view old and current interventions, etc. so that they may be guided accordingly in the care of the patient (Green, 1996).

Another effective technique in communication with the health team is the case conference. This is a regular meeting of all the members of the team wherein they exchange information and plan for the care of the patient. The verbal and written exchange of this conference results in a treatment plan that covers multiple aspects of the patient's care, making sure that the patient is cared for holistically (Kurashi, 2006).

IX. Effective communication in learning about client.

Effective communication can go a long way to helping learn things about the client. It is important to form a good nurse-patient relationship. To effectively communicate with the client to gain her trust as well as gain information about him/her, the nurse must be prepared with information for the client's questions, maintain eye contact, observe body language, listen closely, pay attention to both verbal and non-verbal cues, avoid medical jargon (phrasing questions in ways the patient will understand), and most of all, be sensitive to the client and choose the right moment to ask questions ("Communication skills", 2007).

X. Access to community agencies to meet client needs

As stated above, the home care nurse and the social worker both have access to other community agencies and resources. Through the National Association for Home Care and Hospice, here are some of the affiliates and community agencies that could cater to the needs of the client:

Hospice association of America, Private Duty Homecare Association of America, Center for Health Care Law, World Homecare and Hospice Organization, Pediatric Home Care Association of America, Hospital Home Care Association of America, Proprietary Home Care Association of America, Voluntary Home Care Association of America, Home Medical Equipment Association of America, Psychiatric care services, among others (Kurashi, 2006; "NAHC Affiliates," n.d.)

XI. Organizational and time management techniques for a daily work schedule.

According to Wittenberg (2012), there are many ways to save time for a home health aide:

A. Use time management building blocks:

1. Identify your goals

2. Review your time utilization

3. Match time utilization patterns with your goals

4. Prioritize for better time management

5. Eliminate time bandits (procrastination, perfectionism, etc.)

B. Use computerized documentation

C. Plan and Manage your schedule ahead of time, including your own self-care time

D. Do the whole job, or one thing at a time.

E. Stay focused

F. Telephone management

G. Stress Management.

Bibliography

Wittenberg, S. (2012). Effective Time Management. Retrieved from http://nursing.advanceweb.com/Article/Effective-Time-Management-3.aspx

Davila, L. (n.d.). How to become a Home Health Aide. Retrieved from http://www.innerbody.com/careers-in-health/how-to-become-a-home-health-aide.html

NAHC Affiliates. (2012). Retrieved from http://www.nahc.org/affiliates/home.html

Communication Skills. (2007, Dec 13). *Nursing Times.* Retrieved from http://www.nursingtimes.net/nursing-practice/clinical-zones/educators/communication-skills-essence-of-care-benchmark/361127.article

Schreiner, E. (n.d.). 5 steps to the communication process in the workplace. Retrieved from http://smallbusiness.chron.com/5-steps-communication-process-workplace-16735.html

Communication with patients who have speech and language difficulties. (2009). Retrieved from http://www.patientprovidercommunication.org/article_2.htm

Green, K. (1996). *Home health aide training manual.*
Burlington, MA: Jones & Barlett Learning.

Kurashi, N. (2006). Home health care team members.
Middle East Journal of Age and Ageing, 3(1).
Retrieved from http://www.me-
jaa.com/mejaa6/homehealth.htm

SAMPLE HOME HEALTH AIDE QUESTIONS

1) ……………..provides assistance to the chronically ill, the elderly, and family caregivers who need relief from the stress of care-giving?

    A) Home health Aids

    B) Pastors

    C) Engineers

    D) Surgeons

2) Agencies pay home health aides from payments they receive from the following payers:

    A) Insurance companies

    B) Health maintenance organizations

    C) Medicare

    D) All of the above

3) The Centre for Medicare and Medicaid services payment system for home care is called the:

    A) Home health prospective payment system

    B) Pay per charge

    C) Service payment

    D) Medical payment

4) Clients who need home care are referred by a doctor to a:

    A) Hospital

    B) Friend

    C) Neighbor

D) Home health agency

5) All home health aides are under supervision of one of the following skilled professionals:

A) An engineer

B) A pastor

C) A registered nurse

D) Native medicine

6) All of the following constitute the team of health professionals except:

A) Home health aides

B) Nurses

C) Doctors

D) Engineers

7) ………………helps clients learn to compensate for disabilities:

A) A client

B) An occupational therapist

C) Speech language pathologist

D) Registered dietitian

8) A legal term that means someone can be held responsible for harming someone else is referred to as:

A) Assets

B) Liability

C) Action

D) Discipline

9) A particular method, or way, of doing something is called:

A) Orientation

B) A procedure

C) An activity

D) Information

10) A professional relationship with a client includes:

A) Maintaining a negative attitude

B) Not finishing assignments

C) Doing only the tasks assigned

D) None of the above

11) Professionalism means:

A) Having to do with work or a job

B) Your life outside your job

C) Disapproving client's opinion

D) Keeping late to work

12) ....teaches clients and their families about special diets to improve their health and help them manage their illness:

A) A medical social worker

B) A registered dietitian

C) An occupational therapist

D) None of the above

13) A professional relationship with an employer does not include of the following:

A) Always being on time

B) Completing assignments efficiently

C) Maintaining a negative attitude

D) Participating in education programs offered

14) Which of the following depicts the meaning of laws?

 A) Laws are rules set by the government

 B) Laws tell us what we must do

 C) Laws help to ensure order and safety

 D) All of the above

15) ....defines the things you are allowed to do and describes how to do them correctly:

 A) A plan

 B) A liability

 C) A procedure

 D) A scope of practice

16) Which of the following is not an example of legal and ethical behavior by HHAs?

 A) Protecting client's privacy

 B) Accepting gifts and tips

 C) Being honest at all times

 D) Documenting accurately and promptly

17) Clients have the right to:

 A) Have access, upon request, to all bills for service the client has received

 B) Receive care of the highest quality

 C) Refuse services without fear of reprisal

 D) All of the above

18) Unexplained injuries including burns, bruises, and bone injuries can be referred to as:

 A) Mental abuse

 B) Physical abuse

C) Psychological abuse

D) Passive neglect

19) You can help protect your client's rights in which of the following ways:

A) Respect your clients' property

B) Talk or gossip about a client

C) Neglect clients in your planning

D) Enter a client's room without knocking and seeking permission

20) To respect confidentiality means:

A) To tell the a client's best friend about his friend's health condition

B) To keep private things secret

C) To discuss issues about a client with in a family meeting

D) None of the above

CHAPTER TWO

Medical and social needs of home care clients.

Outline.

1. Introduction

2. Basic physical and emotional needs of clients

3. Recognizing the role of HHA

4. Relating client and family rights to Maslow's hierarchy of needs

5. Culture, lifestyle and life experiences

6. Common reactions to illness/disability

7. Description of basic body functions and changes that should be reported

8. Diseases and disorders common in the healthcare clients

9. Common emotional and spiritual needs

10. Conclusion

Medical and social needs of home care clients.

1. Introduction.

The home health aide has the role of assisting the client and family in managing the condition of health at the clients home. This chapter will describe the needs of the clients, explain the role of the home health aide and relate the rights of the client and family to Maslow's hierarchy of needs. It will also discuss culture, life style and experiences of clients while identifying common reaction to illness or disability, outline body functions, diseases and disorders and emotional or spiritual needs of patients.

2. Basic physical and emotional needs of clients.

Home health aides help clients who have diverse needs so that they feel comfortable and obtain assistance. They include the elderly, infants, mentally ill, people with physical and developmental disabilities together with people with nutritional needs. Majority of the clients require physical assistance in form of service. They often require to be bathed, dressed and given a hand to conduct self-grooming. The client needs to be assisted to wash their hands and perform hygienic tasks to control infections. They need someone to support them as they manage pain. The urinal system may be causing incontinence and they will need someone to help them (Harris, 2004, p. 5).

Clients may have nutritional requirements. The home health aide will assist in making the right combination of food and serve them. Those with skin ailments or wounds require help to take care of the skin and the wounds. The home health aide may be required to change the dressing at the right time. It is within the scope of home health aides to change simple dry dressings, however more complex dressing changes would require a licensed nurse. The disabled and the elderly may have musculoskeletal system problem. They will need someone to assist them in mobility. The bedridden will require someone who understands the best position when turning them in bed or moving them to another location. The HHA will give a hand in ambulation and motion. The client will be in need of a safe environment, the home health aide makes the environment safe for the client. They can clean and arrange their house (Eldelman and Madle 2010, p. 22).

As an important member of the home health team, the HHA is involved in organizing and arranging appointments for the client. Organizing entails arranging the means of transport and accompanying the client to their appointments. At times, she/he assists in doing shopping and cooking appropriate food for the client. They provide company for the client, they keep track of medication taken and appointments with the doctors, they also facilitate the client to participate in certain activities as well as exercise.

Because they work under the supervision of a registered nurse, the home health aides are required to report on the progress of their client. They can be shown how to check respiration rate and temperature for the purpose of helping in a patient's assessment. They follow the care plan in assisting the client with medication reminders to ensure that the client is complying with the medication regimen. According to Ahroni (1989, p. 77), the client needs to be assisted in lifting and coordinating activities. They need someone to provide physical and emotional company. They call in for help in case of emergencies.

Clients in home health care need emotional support from the home health aide. This can be achieved if they talk to them, share stories, read books, and listen to them. Emotional support is needed by the client as they cope with their condition and situation. The family too, needs emotional support. Families living with the mentally ill patients, disabled and terminally ill need encouragement. The new born can be delicate to handle and people may not be sure how to treat them. The caregivers for the infant may have physical and mental constrains. Emotional support also includes taking the client for recreational activities, walking and accompanying them when they ask.

3. Recognizing the roles of HHA.

Home health aides have the responsibility of ensuring that the client is safe and receives adequate care according to the agreement between the home health agency and the family. Every home care client reserves the same patient's rights as those being cared for in the hospital.

The client or family has the right to be involved when the treatment is being planned. They should be given adequate information on the available services and plans as well as how to gain access or terminate the services. The criteria for eligibility should be clearly outlined. The patient should be made aware of their responsibilities. Services provided should be safe and appropriate. The services should also comply with current medical information. Communication should be efficient to allow the patient know when there are changes in service, schedule and medication.

The patient and their family require to be given respect and privacy by the home health aide. The medical information should be kept confidential. The client and their family should not be exploited, mistreated or made uncomfortable. The home health aide can develop a disciplined way of dealing with the patient. For instance, they should avoid yelling, smoking, or ignoring the patient. The patient should be informed about changes in payment when payment is adjusted. The information should be given in advance before changes are made.

Another role of the home health aide is giving quality healthcare. They should respond to the patient's queries appropriately and in time. Services should be of good quality and should be available when required. Quality of health care is informed by healthcare standards and regulations.

In case the patient's status is not improving the home health aide should ensure that they report the progress of the client to the appropriate institution in time. They should be prepared to support and assist the client in the case of emergency. They should inform the patient and family on the necessary procedure and what has caused the action. It is the home health aide duty to ensure they make arrangement together with the patient or family to have the appropriate resources needed. When any service is beyond the scope of the HHA, the registered nurse, usually called the case manager should be informed.

In the case of absenteeism, the home health aide should inform the home health agency, patient or family in advance. They should be cleared if they have terminated the services, are on leave or will come after some time. The home health aide should cooperate and partner with the client and family to provide care. They should not be discriminatory about their religion, culture, gender or race. Being in constant contact with patient gives them the opportunity to establish a relationship with the client to create a good avenue for bringing in emotional and physical support.

4. **Relating client and family rights to Maslow's hierarchy of needs.**

Maslow's hierarchy of needs is an analysis of human needs. Maslow proposes that people chase the fundamental needs first and proceed to successive needs to form a hierarchy (Maslow, 1970, p. 37). When self-actualization needs are met, the person is believed to have acquired growth. Satisfaction of needs is attained as level in hierarchy is accomplished. Therefore, the bottom level in the hierarchy contains the most important needs, while the highest level contains the less important needs. The first level at the bottom of the hierarchy is the physiological level. It entails needs such as water, food, rest, sleep and sex. The client and their family in home care are entitled to the basic needs related to homeostasis. The client, whether elderly, disabled, convalescent or infant should be entitled to access the required food, clean water, and get assisted incase their condition requires oxygen administration. Those are basic requirements for sustenance of life.

The second level from the bottom of the hierarchy is the safety level. The safety needs include: health, environmental safety, availability of resources and employment. The clients and their families have the right to enjoy good health. They have a right to secure environment and not to be exposed to danger. The availability of resources enhances the security of the client and their family. Clients have a need to restore their health and live without ailments. In case they are infants and disabled, they need to be prevented from exposure that could lead to poor health, injuries, sickness or harm. The family and client need medication and a safe environment where they can be comfortable and secure. They need to be assured that procedures and services offered when receiving home health care are safe

The third level from the bottom of hierarchy is the belonging level. People have a desire to feel that they have friends, feel loved and belong to a family. The family of the client should be encouraged to give support to the client. Emotional support from the home health aide will facilitate the feeling of belonging to the client and the family. The client and the family have a right to express and to be shown love. Every human being is entitled to be treated with respect and dignity. Politeness should be exercised when dealing with the client and family.

The fourth level is called self-esteem. Esteem needs include respect, accomplishment, self-esteem and confidence. The client and the family need to experience respect from the home health care team. The home health aide must exercise reverence as they give service. Insult, disrespect and lack of kindness could be considered a violation of their rights. When respect is not granted the patient may lack confidence and loose self-esteem. Maintaining self-esteem will provide a platform for giving emotional support. Esteem is one of the important needs when it comes to mental, physical, social and emotional needs.

The topmost level is self-actualization. The needs are reflected on morality, ability to make decisions and renewal of mind. Morality and ethical considerations of the client and family must be considered. There are professional ethics and laws that are provided for the home health care which must be observed. The home health aide will provide all the information concerning the treatment plan, condition of the client's health, and notify them when there is change in schedule, treatment or payment. The home health aide will ensure that they do not withhold important information on emergency or change in health that requires immediate attention.

5. Culture, lifestyle and life experiences.

Understanding the culture, experience and lifestyle of the client and family will enable the home health aide learn the preferences and attitudes when giving their service. Belonging to a specific community, religion, or any group of people is not a good way of establishing the reasons for the client and their family's behavior. Decision making should be based on their choices and attitude.

Culture, lifestyle and life experience dictates what values the client and the family has. It is necessary to observe the relationship of the client and their family. Cultural values could affect choices of health in different patients. For instance, some ailments or disability may be associated with negative meaning. People vary in experience because they grow up and live in diverse regions. Understanding their lifestyle could give ideas if their ailment could have been caused by their choice of lifestyle. Cultural values could give ideas on how to treat an elderly person. Furthermore, it will give information on the kind of language to be used. This could bring in new ideas like introducing an interpreter. It is not advisable to touch every object one sees in a client's home as some objects may hold sacred significance. When a HHA is assigned to a client, it is the professional duty of the HHA to familiarize themselves with the family. For example, ask how the client prefers to be addressed. For some individuals, addressing them by their first name or other pet names like *honey* or *sweetie* may be insultive.

Wernig and Sorrentine (1989, p. 81) note that people value culture and respect it. Culture is the sum total of the way of life of an individual or a group of people. The home health aide should show respect to the client's culture and desist from *ethnocentrism* which means thinking that one's culture is superior to another person's culture. The more respect and cultural diversity observed, the more comfortable the client and their family will be with the agency. Failure to recognize their cultural values and beliefs could lead to mistrust. Obviously, this can be avoided. The home health aide can engage into a relationship with the client and the family to find out what their feelings are and if they are exercising any fear about the client's condition. Treating a person with dignity and giving quality care could be seen as a significant way of giving value to the client. Identifying cultural prejudices is an effective way of becoming culturally aware. When one pays attention to their beliefs and cultural practices, they choose to adjust their behavior to treat them right. It is very easy to say to oneself "I respect other people's culture, this section of the book is not for me". But take time to ask your self the following questions:

1. How do I feel when someone who has a different accent speaks to me?

2. Do I feel my food is superior when I perceive the odor of foods from other cultures?

3. Do other people's dressing make me uncomfortable?

4. Do I feel people do not know what they believe just because they do not believe in my own God?

Depending on an individual's culture, lifestyle and experience, the home health aide should assess beliefs about sickness and death. They contribute to understanding attitude towards health, attitude on the service of the home health aide, alternative ways of gaining health, religious beliefs, family influence, communication and the client's opinion about their health. Because of lifestyle and life experience, the client and family may have perceptions about medical care and home healthcare aides.. They may have negative or positive experience with the healthcare system. Negative experience could cause a client who is elderly or disabled refuse to cooperate. One can also establish the decision making of the family. There are cases where the family male head makes decision, while in other families members discuss and give a common answer. The client may be able to give their decisions and they should be considered. Matters of religion can play a major role in the way the client and family perceives illness. While some may reject some treatment and choose other alternatives, others believe in supernatural power of healing. Depending on experience and culture, clients and family will have diverse response to the home health care. In order to explain the effect of culture on illness, let me discuss a bit about the Igbo culture in Nigeria, West Africa.

The Igbo Culture

The Igbo people usually called 'Ibo' by non-Igbos are situated in the southeast region of Nigeria in West Africa. The area is divided by the Niger River into two unequal sections – the eastern region which is the larger part, and the Midwestern region. The global health case study states that 'According to Nigeria's National Census (1991), the Igbo cultural group accounted for 25 million of the 88.9 million people in the country' .The population reference bureau updates that Nigerian population had increased to 140 million in 2006, and the southern states of which the Igbos constitute a large part of accounted for 65 million. The Igbos speak the Igbo language, and they have two major religions : Christianity and traditional religion. Christianity is the belief in Jesus as the son of God, and Lord, while their traditional religion is the worship of idols, believing that many of the idols are small gods that point to 'Chukwu' meaning the big God. The Igbos are known to value education, hence in present day Igbo culture, the minimum education one would have is the high school certificate. Actually high school graduates are considered illiterates.

Their staple food is 'Garri' which is processed from cassava. It could be drunk as a cereal, or baked into cakes. But the most common way of eating it is to make it as a dough, and eat it with different kinds of soups. Mostly vegetable packed soups. Other staple foods are Rice and Yam, to name a few. The cultural practices of the Igbos include: 'The new yam festival' which is usually celebrated around October of every year when the new yam is harvested; 'Igba Nkwu Nwanyi' meaning pouring wine for the bride. This is the name given to their costly marriage ceremony, where the groom has to spent the savings of a long period to get married. This usually contributes to the longevity of the Igbo marriages, if unfaithfulness is noted or other conflicts, and the lady decides to go home to her parents, another ceremony is performed. This practice has helped couples to resolve their differences on time before it gets out hand. Of course there are several other practices which the scope of this paper will constrain me to write.

The health beliefs of this ethnic group in relation to health and illness include the following:

- That most illnesses are caused by one's enemies who submitted their names to evil sprits.
- That some illnesses are a reward of one's evil doing in the past.
- That evil spirits could be appeased to cure mysterious illnesses.
- That health is a gift from God (Chukwu) and should be maintained by good food, so the eating of fruits and vegetables is usually the norm, as these vegetables are mostly grown from family gardens and are not bought in the market. Even if they are bought, they are very affordable.
- That husbands should stick to their wives sexually to prevent 'Nsi Nwanyi' meaning myserious illness gotten

from women. This is the common name for sexually transmitted diseases.

- The use of local herbs to cure illnesses which have been proven to be effective over the ages.

The specific health and illness needs of the Igbo people include:

- Lack of portable drinking water: Water is usually bought from some rich people that installed bore-hole systems. The public tap water which is the main source of water supply is not usually maintained by the government because of misappropriation of funds. This water problem is usually worse during the dry season, because during the rainy season. The source of water supply is usually Rainfall.

- Most families are low income earners and the staple foods which are garri, yam and rice are usually costly. So under nourishment is usually a problem which could be solved by the assisted nutritional services like food stamps or free food programs.

- The main disease or illness suffered by this group is Malaria. But there have been many resources and curative measures available, so mortality from malaria is almost a thing of the past.

- According to a global health case study, 'Agriculture is a heritage occupation and remains quite traditional with small sized farms, and rain-fed crop production. All crops cultivated are used as food. Nonetheless, both protein-energy and micronutrient deficiencies are a public health problem'.

- Over-crowding is a major problem as people are over crowded in cars, schools, and living places. This usually aids in the transmission of infectious diseases easily.

- Majority of the Igbo people suffer from and die from stroke since healthcare is not affordable for early diagnoses of the illness. And to make it worse, when somebody slumps on the way in a real village setting, no help is called for as it is believed that the evil spirits tormenting the individual would start tormenting the helper. This is recently improving with the continuous health education on heart attacks, and strokes.

Road traffic accidents (RTA) is one of the major causes of death in this area, because of lack of proper driving regulations. A health education research supports this by stating that 'Data taken from admissions records to the hospital and private clinics (the three facilities which treat accidents) show a similar dominance of RTAs. All entries relating to unintentional injuries were extracted for 1 year, from March 1993 to March 1994. Ninety-nine entries were recorded, of which 63 were injuries caused by RTAs'.

Their ways of meeting healthcare needs include the following:

- Since there is no health insurance, and health delivery is usually based on availability of cash payment by the patient, people usually go to the hospital when they are really sick. This aids in a high rate of mortality level because in some cases, the illnesses are at their end stage.

- Thanks to the government of the Igbo people that both over the counter drugs and prescriptions drugs can be gotten over the counter even with no prescription. And medications are sold relatively cheap, far cheaper than that what hey are sold here in the United States. Hence antibiotics, anti-malarial drugs, and most common diseases can be easily bought, and

48

one follows the dosage on the drugs. If not for this, millions of people would have died because they could not afford hospital bills.

- Many deliveries are done by experienced traditional midwives or people that have have some background in healthcare, and this is done either in their homes, or in their some small private clinics. This reduces the cost of child birth, and pregnant mothers are usually referred to the hospitals if their pregnancy is complicated. The negative effect is that many babies are lost, and some mothers do not make it to the hospital.

- Apart from traditional midwives helping in deliveries, they also help in circumcision of males. There are also herbalists that are known and proven to use herbs to cure illnesses.

- Some herbs like 'Akum, shut up!' are grown by most people in their back yard. 'Akum' means malaria, shut up is an English language. This herb is very bitter, but when soaked in water and drunk, cures malaria. Keep in mind that malaria is the commonest illness in this culture, although the fatality has greatly reduced because of availability of its cure in various ways.

Some areas of conflict between cultural practices and the healthcare delivery system include the following:

- The strong belief that one's illness is caused by one's enemies prevents people from seeking healthcare delivery, because it is believed to be useless in such cases. Many people die because of this belief.

- The smuggling in of herbal preparations into the hospitals usually affects real assessment of the success of the treatment plan. Usually nurses make it a routine to search patients' surroundings to make sure that there are no hidden preparations.

- Some people do not want to be blamed for not going to the hospital, so they go, but cheek their medications, and throw them away when the nurse leaves the room, fake recovery after a few two or three days from admission, and go home. This could either be from believing in a non-scientific origin of the illness, or other personal beliefs.

- It is usually a thing of pride to have a non-eventful pregnancy, which is crowned by a vaginal delivery of the baby. Hence many women try everything they can to have vaginal delivery to maintain their ego, as people who have not gone through normal delivery and gone through the pains of childbirth are not 'real women'. Some end up losing their babies or their lives in the process of being 'real women'. The home health aide should practice attentive listening to understand why the client believes in what they hold fast. Personal biases should be relegated to the side.

6. Common reactions to illness/disability.

It is important for the home health aide student to be prepared in dealing with the reaction of the client and family on their condition or illness. The elderly, convalescent, disabled and infants may not be able to perform certain duties. Additionally, their condition may not allow them to generate income. This means that they are dependent on others for service and financial support. If the financial burden is very high on the family, family constraints can occur. Some families have insurance and get the relief.

Some family members may not be willing to give service, for fear of contracting the disease or other reasons like dedication to job or just not being able to cope with the stress of a loved one that is dependent. The burden of taking care of the client may be left to one person. As the family

51

gives support to the client, they develop emotional, psychological and physical needs. They may end up with limited time to take care for themselves.

The challenge emerging from the home health care can cause depression to the patient and family. Demands for more resources and time can be tiring. Moreover, taking care of the patient could be very demanding and cause stress. If the patient does not show any improvement after the services of the home health agency have been employed, anxiety may crop in for lack of progress. They may live in worry; lose self-esteem and start experiencing moments of grief because of client's condition. If stress on the part of the client and their family is not managed well they could end up in destructive behaviors. The client may attempt to withhold from treatment, the family may ignore their responsibility and become hostile or on the other extreme, become over-protective. Home health environment where working relations are constrained and the family is fully or partially withdrawn from giving support may become stressed. Good relationship between a client and their family facilitate creating a complimentary environment for home care.

Assessing the needs of the client and that of the family will inform the plan when giving service. The home health aide should evaluate the most important and the less significant needs and give priority according to the needs. It is necessary to give the family and the client relevant information that can help them cope with the situation. Getting them to increase their knowledge about the circumstances will give them a reason for negative reactions. Family members who feel overburdened by the demands of the resources could seek alternatives such as insurance. They can be referred to a program that educates and provides support for people with similar health needs. In the case where one of the family members is overburdened with responsibilities, arrangements can be made to reduce the burden. The family can request support from other family members to get economic relief resulting from the conditions of the client. There is need to treat depression and stress to facilitate good health. Training on how to deal with the special need of the client can be given. Engaging in a program will facilitate an opportunity for the family and client to share with others and reduce the chances of getting stressed (Doenges et al, 2010, p. 67).

7. Description of basic body functions and changes that should be reported.

Basic body functions can be explained by understanding the functions of the organs of the body. The integumentary system is responsible for normalizing temperature of the body, generate hormones and support the sensory organs. Skeletal system facilitates body movements, stores blood cells and minerals. Muscular organs give the body posture, warmth and enables movement. The nervous system enables communication and control between the surrounding and the body. Endocrine body functions include generation and distribution of hormones to the blood. Circulatory system distributes immunity and required substances to different parts of the body. The lymphatic system facilitates transportation of fluids in the body.

The respiratory system basic function is to excrete carbon dioxide and inhale oxygen. The digestion enables the body transform food into nutrients and excretes the unwanted waste from the body. Urinary organs remove waste, and create a balance between acid and electrolytes with water. Reproductive organs are responsible for generating sex cells and allowing transfer as well as fertilization to produce new offspring.

The home health aide should ensure that they report any changes that threaten the life of the client. This may include persistent respiratory difficulties, frequent falls and reduced level of consciousness that cannot be explained. They should report when the blood sugar is very high despite medication. Similarly, very high blood pressure or very low blood pressure. Drug reactions must also be reported for the physician to make adjustments. The home health aide should make it a routine to report to the home health care agency the client's progress (Birchenall, 2012, p. 61).

8. Diseases and disorders common in the healthcare clients.

There are diseases and disorders that HHAs should be aware of because they are common in home health care. The elderly people complain of Dementia. Dementia is characterized by impaired cognition and loss of memory. The elderly demonstrates neurological disorders. Neurological disorders signs can include pain in the muscle especially when making movement. The elderly may suffer from incontinence. Symptoms of incontinence are loss of control of bladder.

Another common disease in the elderly is cardiovascular disease. Some may experience a heart attack, cardiac arrest or high blood pressure. The Arthritis is another disease common in home care. Signs of arthritis include pain in the ankle, knee, feet, wrist, hip, hands, back, spine, neck and shoulder. Elderly have challenges with their vision and earring. Their vision becomes blurred and they may require one to talk aloud enough so that they can hear (Shouting is avoided). The vision problems could have been caused by glaucoma or muscular degeneration. Some elderly clients have diabetes. Signs and symptoms include blood glucose that is high, sweating and blurred visions. Some have sleeping disorders.

The elderly may have osteoporosis. Osteoporosis makes bones break easily and takes a long time to heal, and cause injuries and sprains. Other clients may have lung disease, which causes them to breath with difficulty. Skin disorders are common in home health care. Skin disorder signs include irritation of the skin, rashes and sensitive skin (Sommers, 2010, p. 25).

Cancer is another disease prevalent in home care. Cancer is an abnormal proliferation of cells can affect any part of the body. In any cancerous cell, there is growth without control. There are various forms of cancer, others are gender based. The client could suffer from cognitive disorders. It could be in for of delirium syndrome. The symptoms include disturbed conscience, disorganized thoughts and agitation.

9. Common emotional and spiritual needs.

A terminally ill client together with their family has different emotional and spiritual needs. They have different abilities to cope with the situation. While some may be in denial, others may have accepted reality. Majority of the terminally ill patient go through the grieving process. They first deny the news and isolate themselves. They experience anger and strong emotions of despair. They quickly realize the reality and begin to bargain on the life in their thoughts. They then enter into a depression. Finally, they accept the reality and begin to give their best in the remaining days. The home health aide understands that the family undergoes Kubler-Ross stages of grief which has the acronym: DABDA. D-Denial, A-Anger, B-Bargaining, D-Depression, A-Acceptance.

The terminally ill and the family agonize and feel pain for the anticipated loss. The terminally ill experiences pain from the illness. They have feelings of helplessness for not being able to accomplish all they wanted in life. The patient may go into depression because they are not able to meet their responsibilities. The family members become depressed after seeing that they cannot restore the health of their loved one (Birchenall and Streight, 2003, p. 11).

The interventions for emotions include allowing the patient and the family talk to a therapist or counselor about their experience. One can facilitate and organize for the family to spend a lot of time with each other. They can be encouraged to share their thoughts and feelings. In their discussion they can be helped to deal with anxiety and fear.

This can be done by showing them how to relax. They can exercise breathing exercise. Their concerns on medication and treatment for comfort should be conversed. Allowing the client time to express their feelings is very important. Bottled emotions do not help with coping. Venting emotions helps to relax the muscles and helps client to explore ways that can serve as coping strategies.

Spiritual support involves inviting the client's religious leader for spiritual guidance. The client and family can be encouraged to get the support from their clergy. Interacting with the clergy will create avenues for asking questions and obtaining answers about spiritual matters. The religious leader can provide spiritual support which is effective in dealing with anxiety (Stanworth, 2003, p. 30).

10. Conclusion.

The client needs someone to help them bath, dress do self-grooming, control infections, take medication, get help in mobility, manage pain, safe environment and get help with cleaning. They need company and encouragement as emotional support. The home health aide should follow the care plan in providing service. The client and family, just like every other individual follow Maslow's hierarchy of needs which include the physiological, safety, belonging, esteem and self-actualization needs. Culture, lifestyle and experience of client and family motivate their decision making and perception about the condition of the client. Illnesses and disability cause financial constraints and need for service. Support helps the client and family deal with constraints. Changes such as unconsciousness, persistent high blood sugar and persistent difficulty in breathing should be reported. Many clients in home care have Dementia, neurological disorders, incontinence, cardiovascular disease, arthritis, poor vision, hearing difficulties, diabetes, osteoporosis, sleeping disorders, cancer and cognitive disorders. The client and family need encouragement when the patient is terminally ill. They can be given support by their religious leaders.

Bibliography

Ahroni, J. H. (1989). A description of the health needs of the elderly home care patients with   chronic illness. *Home Health Care Service Quarterly,* 10, 3, 77-92.

Birchenall, J. M. (2012). Mosby's Textbook for the Home Aide. New Jersey: Mosby.

Birchenall, J. M., and Streight, E. (2003) Mosby's Textbook for the Homecare aide, 2nd edition,   New Jersey: Mosby.

Doenges, M., Moorhouse,M., and Murr, A. (2010) Nurse's   Pocket   Guide: Diagnoses,   Prioritized   Interventions and Rationales.   Philadelphia: F.A. Davis Company.

Eldelman, C. L., and Madle, C. L. (2010). Health promotion   throughout   the   Life   span,   seventh   edition. New Jersey: Mosby.

Harris, M. D. (2004). Handbook of Home Health Care Administration. London: Jones & Bartlett   Publishers.

Maslow, A. H. (1970). Motivation and personality, 2nd edition., New York: Harper and Row.

Sommers, M. (2010) Diseases and Disorders: A Nursing Therapeutics Manual. Philadelphia: F.A. Davis Company.

Stanworth, R. (2003) Recognizing Spiritual Needs in People who are Dying. Oxford: OUP   Oxford.

Wernig, J. K., and Sorrentine, S. A. (1989). Homemaker-Home Health Aide. *Journal of Health   Occupation and Education*, 5, 1, 81-82.

SAMPLE HOME HEALTH AIDE QUESTIONS

21) ………………..is the process of exchanging information with others:

A) Looking

B) Recreation

C) Communication

D) Interpretation

22) Always report combative behaviors of clients to your:

A) Parents

B) Client's friend

C) Friend

D) Supervisor

23) All of the following are some barriers to communication, except:

A) Client hears and understands you clearly

B) Client is difficult to understand

C) Asking why

D) Client speaking in a different language

24) Which of the following questions would you ask a client for adequate clarifications?

A) Did you sleep last night?

B) Did he rape you?

C) Tell me about your sleep last night

D) Is exercise good?

25) Reasons for documentation include:

A) It guarantees clear and complete communication

B) It provides up-to-date record of the status of a client

C) Documentation protects you and the employer from liability

D) All of the above

26) File an incident report when one of the following incidents occurs:

A) You client performs an exercise

B) Your client falls

C) When a patient is safe

D) When a client lies on the right side of the body

27) The process of removing pathogens or state of being free from pathogens is referred to as:

A) Medical asepsis

B) Plasmodiasis

C) Sepsis

D) Toxoplasmosis

28) …………..is where the pathogen lives and grows:

A) House

B) Ecosystem

C) Landscape

D) Reservoir

29) An uninfected person who could get sick or infected is referred to as a:

A) Portal of entry

B) Causative agent

C) Susceptible host

D) Sepsis

30) If blood or body fluid spills on fabrics such as carpets and clothes:

A) Use alcohol to clean it

B) Use commercial disinfectants to clean it

C) Clean with bleach

D) None of the above

31) ....is a federal government agency that issues information to protect the health of individuals and communities:

A) Health firm

B) World health organization

C) The centre for disease control and prevention

D) Individual co-operations

32) One of the following is not included as one of the measures of standard precautions:

A) Clean a client's blood without wearing gloves

B) Wash your hands before putting on gloves

C) Wear gloves if you may come in contact with body fluids

D) Wear a disposable gown that is resistant to body fluid

33).....................refers to washing hands with water and soap or other detergents that contain an antiseptic agent:

  A) Hand antisepsis

  B) Hand rinsing

  C) Protocols

  D) None of the above

34) Equipment that helps protect employees from serious injuries or illnesses resulting from contact with workplace hazards is called:

  A) Personal protective equipment

  B) Standard precaution

  C) Hospital policy

  D) Health machineries

35) Personal protective equipment includes the following, except one:

  A) Masks

  B) Goggles

  C) Gowns

  D) Needles

36) One of the following is not an airborne disease:

  A) Measles

  B) Tuberculosis

  C) Boil

  D) Chickenpox

37) Droplets can be created by:

  A) Coughing

  B) Sneezing

C) Laughing

D) All of the above

38) An example of a droplet disease is the:

A) Rash

B) Scabies

C) Mumps

D) Constipation

39) MRSA stands for:

A) Menstrual reluctant stage of Action

B) Men Rehabilitation system activities

C) Methicillin-resistant staphylococcus aureas

D) None of the above

40) Droplet precautions include:

A) Wearing a face mask during care

B) Restricting visits from uninfected people

C) An infected client covering his nose and mouth with a tissue when sneezing

D) All of the above

41) The way the parts of the body works together whenever you move is referred to as:

A) Body mechanics

B) Movement

C) Body structure

D) Matrix

42) When you stand, your weight is centered in:

A) Elbows

B) Your arms

C) Your pelvis

D) Fibula

43) Disorientation means confusion about:

A) Person

B) Place

C) Time

D) All of the above

44) Burns can be caused by one of the following:

A) Cold water

B) Hand shaking

C) Dry heat

D) Waxing floors

45) Employee's responsibilities for infection control include the following:

A) Follow standard precautions

B) Take advantage of the free hepatitis B vaccination

C) Immediately report any exposure you have to infection, or blood

D) All of the above

46) One of the following is not a guideline to guide against fire:

A) Stay in or near the kitchen when anything is cooking

B) Discourage careless smoking and smoking in bed

C) Turn on heaters when no one is home

D) Do not leave dryer on when you leave the house

47) To ensure travel safety:

A) Avoid planning your route

B) Use turn signals

C) Encourage distractions from friends

D) Drive without seat belt

48) Factors that raise the risk for falls include:

A) Clutter

B) Slippery floors

C) Poor lighting

D) All of the above

49) …………..is emergency care given immediately to an injured person?

A) Exercise

B) Head stretching

C) 9111

D) First aid

50) The first signs of insulin reaction include one of the following:

A) Pneumonia

B) Heart failure

C) Constipation

D) Nervousness

CHAPTER THREE

Personal Care Services by the Home Health Aide

Outline

1. Introduction

2. Steps and guidelines for common personal care

3. Importance of improvising equipment and adapting care activities in the home

4. Personal care delivery at home

5. Examples of equipment that can be used to provide care

6. Benefits of self-care in promoting wellness

7. Key principles of body mechanics

8. How to adapt body mechanics in the home

9. Adaptations that can be made in the home for ambulation and positioning

10. The purpose of passive and active range motion exercise

11. High risk factors for skin breakdown and methods of prevention

12. Stages of pressure ulcers/decubitus ulcers and report observation

13. Types of ostomies and how to empty and change the pouch

14. Emergencies in the home and critical steps to follow

15. The chain of infection to the home care setting

16. Infection control measures to use in the home care setting

17. Role and responsibilities of the HHA in assisting the client to self-administer medications

18. Conclusion

Personal Care Services by the Home Health Aide

1. Introduction.

Personal care is important in the management of home care clients. Personal care enables the client to feel comfortable and prevent other illnesses. This chapter will discuss personal care, equipment needed and taking care of the skin. It will also talk about infection and the role of home health aide in self-administered medications.

2. Steps and guidelines for common personal care.

The client in need of home healthcare usually requires assistance in personal care. The home health aide should have skills such as bed bath, tub bathing and shower bathing. They should be very familiar with the guidelines of transferring or lifting the client when they want to change position. Personal care skills will also include lifting the patient from the floor. The personal care skills are necessary because the client may not be able to move independently. Their mobility can be limited because they suffered from a stroke that may have caused brain damage, body weakness or caused them to have unusual posture. Correct steps in personal care eases positioning and transfer as well as, maintains comfort for the client. The steps and guidelines in personal care assist in fostering safety when moving the client. The client and the home health aide reduce the chances of injury when conducting personal care. (Birchenall 2012, p. 33)

A bed bath is refreshing, allows skin inspection and allows change of beddings. A bed bath begins with ensuring privacy, informing the client of the intention of bath and maintaining a good conversation. The home health aide should prepare for bath by ensuring the room temperature is warm, door is closed, window and curtains are pulled for confidentiality. Collect all the equipment and materials to include: big pan or bowl, two firm chairs, soap and soap dish, bathing cloth, towels, a plastic covering for protection of chair from becoming wet and preferred cloths. The two chairs can be placed next to the bed, and then one chair is covered with the plastic covering. The soap, dish and big pan are placed on the covered chair. The other chair is for placing the beddings. Light covers can be left to make the bed have warmth. The client can be requested to cooperate or assist in removing cloths, from top to bottom. The top can be cleaned, dried out and covered with cloths before moving to the bottom. The body parts that are paralyzed should be the last when removing cloths. The bottom cloths should be slipped slowly from waist to knee to the feet, one side first and then the other side if the person is unable to lift weight. Only the areas being cleaned should not be covered. The water in the bowl should be half full and tested with elbow for appropriate temperature. The soap should be kept in the dish and wash cloth used as required (Birchenall and Streight, 2003, p. 66).

To wash the client's face, the neck and bellow should be covered. Dampen cloth and squeeze out water and hold all the edges before cleaning the face without soap unless requested. Then wash the neck and ears with soap and dry. Wash the arms and hands with wet soapy cloth using long strokes. Then clean the abdomen and chest while paying attention to folds especially under the breast. Wash the front and lower part of body with circular movements and then wash the legs. The legs can be elevated for access and used with warm wet and soapy cloth using long strokes. Start with hips to knees and then knees to the feet. The feet can be cleaned while paying attention to in between the toes. If the client is unable they can be assisted to clean perennial area. The client can be helped to sit on a towel, by rolling them to one side . The cloth can be given sparing soap, dampened and squeezed. The client can be given the cloth and allowed to clean self. The home health aide should face away as they clean. If they are unable, one should clean using strokes that start from front to back. Pay attention to skin folds and dry well. Clean the clients back and remaining sides, from top to bottom and apply skin oil or lotion. At this point one can place the linen on the bed when the client is still on the side. The cloths should be worn beginning with the paralyzed body parts from the top to the bottom. The client should be allowed to choose pajamas or clothing.

Guidelines for lifting and transferring propose that the load should be closest to the body as possible. This allows the center of gravity to be close to the support's base. A wide base for support is considered safe. This means that when lifting a load, one can use the surface close to floor with large base for support. Placing the legs apart creates a wide base for support. The back can be kept straight by bending the knee and hips, while lifting load to lower the center of gravity and use the feet instead of the back. Always move the leg when making a turn and avoid twisting, which can be painful or cause injury. Small steps are useful in maintaining a stronger base when moving. When lifting load to a position above the head use a stool to step on. Load above the head lowers the centre of gravity (Wernig and Sorrentine, 1989, p. 81).

3. **Importance of improvising equipment and adapting care activities in the home.**

Depending on the needs of the client Cain (1940, p. 294) suggests that, different equipment may be improvised because of cost and safety in their use. An example is the use of plastic chairs in bathing. The plastic chairs are affordable and easy to maintain clean. The improvised equipment will cut down on cost for extra costs that could have been used to purchase expensive equipment. The comfort of the client is maintained with less costly equipment. The improvised equipment are easy to use and can be applied across all social classes. Improvised equipment are helpful when required equipments are broken or not available. They facilitate the comfort of the client as they receive personalized care. The improvised equipment endorses self-care in the home.

Improvised equipment that can assist in the homecare activities can make a difference in creating good quality of life for the client. The client can gain independence and adapt to changes in their life. Adaptation can make the client feel comfortable and obtain fulfilling personalized care. The patient can sleep well, eat and move in and outside their home when they want.

The availability of improvised equipment and adaptive care activities cause those in need of home health aide come to terms with the progress of their health condition. The activities include rearranging the house for easy mobility and use of when chairs because of weak legs.

The client uses the improvised equipment or adaptive activity because it is necessary.

Adaptive care activities necessitate the home health aide to adjust equipment and activities according to the need of the client. Improvised equipment may become convenient and suitable for client when designed for the need of the patient.

4. Personal care delivery at home.

Personal care delivery at home entails giving personalized care according to individual needs of a client. It encourages comfort and safety to the client as they receive care. Personal care delivery entails giving healthcare services using skills while paying attention to safety and comfort of the client. Using the available information, the home health aide uses appropriate skills to deliver care to the client. They skillfully employ communication skills to facilitate their work. They interact with the patient, family and other healthcare professional to give best care as the client obtains healthcare in their home (Shi and Singh 2011, p. 5).

5. Examples of equipment that can be used to provide care.

Equipment used to provide personalized care include: wheel chair for transportation, mobility aids for clients with weak feet, transferring aids, lifting aids, breathing aids, audio and visual aids, incontinence equipment, beds, feeding aids, Hoyer lifts, diapers,

6. Benefits of self-care in promoting wellness.

Self-care is the involvement of an individual in decisions concerning their health. A person practicing self-care is aware of healthcare needs and makes informed decision. Self-care is characterized by healthy eating habits, appropriate lifestyle preferences and being informed on when to ask for medical assistance. Self-care entails making the appropriate decisions to exercise, take a balanced diet, get enough sleep and being kept to prevent any infections that can harm health. Self-care can cause one to get immunized, treat infections and sickness before it advances, get screening for any conditions for early detection, follow recommended prescription and getting the correct appointment with a physician. Consequently, a client is able to make correct decisions about concerning their health. For instance, a healthy diet will make the body strong and prevent some illnesses caused by deficiency such as anemia. A healthy or balanced diet will keep sickness away. Balanced diet will enable the body to form a strong immune system. Self-care can cause one to choose whether to treat a minor illness at home or at the hospital. It is easy to treat illness when one gives priority to a healthy diet and is able to take their medication as prescribed.

Self-care practices facilitate a good relationship between the client and the healthcare professionals. Communicating with the health care practitioners and the client becomes easier than when the patient is not aware of self-care. Self-care eventually causes one to have good quality of life by preventing and managing illness. Moreover, there is confidence in decision making and hope for improved health (Canadian Pharmacists Association, 2002, p. 5).

7. Key principles of body mechanics.

Body mechanics uses different parts of the body to make safe movement, conserve energy and increase efficiency when conducting different activities with the body. Body mechanics discourage incorrect posture when using the body and reveals physical capabilities.

Body mechanics emphasize balance when performing an action. Unity of action is considered as an important factor in attaining support. All the necessary muscles can be used to give support when a person is moving. The abdomen is considered a powerful source of power. The physical power can also be coordinated with the aid of the abdomen together with the back. The back should be kept upright to give control.

Body mechanics that can be adapted in homecare is to use the correct posture to stand or sit. The chin should be lowed, shoulder rest towards the back and squared. The hips should be above knees when standing up. Twisting should be avoided. When lifting the heavy objects, the muscles in the leg can be used when legs are apart. The knees together with hips should be used for bending while the back is kept straight. The object being should be close to the body. When pulling and pushing, use both hands as well as the legs to acquire force. Use the palm instead of fingers and let the feet be firmly held to the ground when pushing. Pulling and pushing should be preferred to lifting. When reaching out or bending, the feet should be firmly placed on ground and the shoulders apart. The knees can be bending while the hips should be bending slightly. Avoid balancing or step on a higher ground (or stool). Exercising is another principle that can enable the body performs many functions. The abdomen and leg support lifting, pulling and pushing. When the body is flexible bending is easy. The shoulders give the back a support for posture.

Exercising makes the body flexible and strengthens the muscles as Dixon (2000, p. 56) notes.

8. How to adapt body mechanics in the home.

The home health aide can adapt motions that are safe for the client and themselves. This will involve supporting the client when they perform exercise and advice on the safe motions. They may use skills to transfer and lift them. When transferring a client one should ensure that they plan before they act. They should ensure their back is not bending and only lift the person if they are able. They should ask for assistance if the client has a lot of weight. When lowering the client on should spread the legs and avoid twisting.

9. Adaptations that can be made in the home for ambulation and positioning.

The home health aide can ensure that the client gets physical support to sit, stand and move. The client can be supported with pillows when sited. One can hold their hand under the arm and closely to give them support as they stand and walk. Ensure the client changes position after a while to avoid exerting too much pressure on one side.

10. The purpose of passive and active range motion exercise.

Passive range of motions is practiced in clients who cannot do exercise without support. The motions are done with the assistance of a professional to help strengthen muscle and joint with stretching. The purpose of passive range motions is to facilitate gentle movement to muscles and joints for daily movement. The body remains healthy and chances of being completely incapacitated by an illness are lowered. On the other hand, Action range motion exercises are conducted by a health professional to a client who can do exercises without support and therefore only receives instructions for exercising.

Passive and active range motions secure the muscles from atrophy and enhance circulation. After the motions, the client pain alleviates and they become strong. The client benefits from body flexibility after the exercises.

11. High risk factors for skin breakdown and methods of prevention.

The skin forms the largest organ of the body. A third of the blood circulation occurs in the skin. The skin protects the body from heat, physical acts, chemicals and light. Furthermore, the skin shields the body from infection, maintains good environment and is an important sensory organ. Additionally, the skin retains water, vitamin D and fats that are important. The skin is resilient and can heal after an injury.

Besides being resilient, the skin can undergo a breakdown if the following factors are experienced. When the skin is abused for a long time by friction and moisture can breakdown. A lot of pressure and force will damage the skin. Clients with myelitis, paralysis or illness that cause loss of sensation are susceptible to a skin breakdown. Paralysis affects skin tissue; where the collagen is reduced making the skin loses elasticity. Additionally, the muscles do not function and the lack of padding could lead to skin breakdown.

Clients who have difficulty shifting weight lack sensation to be able to adjust their position. Their skin can be exposed to extreme heat, cold, discomfort, trauma or sun for long. The client's skin with impaired sensation can be injured from heat near a fire place or a lap top. Ice packs and extreme cold can cause frost bite. Toe nails can in grow and get infected without the client feeling pain. Skin can get sun burns without the client noticing.

Clients who have impaired sensation and reduced mobility may have pressure ulcers, which is a type of skin breakdown. Other types of skin breakdown reveal as a blister, cut, scrape or burn. Pressure ulcers may affect the bone and sometimes require surgery. Skin break down still occur even when care is taken and is preventable. Prescribed equipment and care does not guarantee that skin breakdown cannot occur. When the skin breakdown occurs care must be given in the initial stages before it advances. Skin breakdown advances from the initial stages to the advanced stages very quickly (Habif et al 2011, p. 9).

Another factor that can cause skin breakdown is poor nutrition and failure to have liquid food or water. In addition, people who are overweight because of pressure on a particular side if unable to move. Clients with depression or those who abuse substances may be unable to attend to their body. Clients with depression may disregard self-care and neglect their skin.

The skin can be kept clean and dry. Mild soaps can be used for bath, with warm water; since hot water can cause skin dryness. When drying the skin, avoid rubbing and use patting technique. The undergarments should be changed frequently. Pads should be changed immediately after bowel. Adapting to a therapy where the client exercises to strengthen muscles, increase circulation and facilitate flexibility is necessary. Skin breakdown can be prevented by feeding on a balanced diet and taking adequate water. Cutting down on weight will reduce body mass that compress blood vessels. Clients can eat foods rich in Omega three, Zinc, Protein, and Vitamins A and C. The foods nourish the sin and prevent skin breakdown.

Prolonged pressure on one side can be eliminated by changing positions often. Change positions in bed after around three hours and place pillows at the back. Avoid sleeping on the back if the client had been using a wheel chair. Ensure the client is able to breathe comfortably at all times. Muscle spasms can be managed to allow control by exercising. Straps or braces should be comfortable to avoid pressure if worn correctly.

12. Stages of pressure ulcers/decubitus ulcers and report observation.

Pressure ulcers are characterized by injury of skin or tissue bellow skin from combined friction and pressure. The home health aide should look at the skin to check to check the condition. There are four stages of skin breakdown. In the first stage the skin changes color to red, blue or grey after close to fifteen minutes without pressure, although the skin is still intact. In the next stage the epidermis together with the dermis layers loses skin thickness. In the following stage, all skin thickness is lost to a depression since the dermis and epidermis layer are absent. In the final and advanced stage the entire skin layers, muscles, bones and tendons are lost. The home health aide can report rashes, turgor, bruises, wrinkles, veins, and bumps. The temperature can be noted whether, cold, warm, cool or hot. Changes that must be reported include: redness or change in skin color, irritation, odor, swelling, drainage, sores and perspiration. It should be reported if the client experiences burning, pain and tingling in the affected skin (Habif 2011, p. 93).

13. Types of ostomies and how to empty and change the pouch.

An ostomy is a surgical opening on a body after a surgery. Types of ostomies include: Colostomy, ileostomy and Urostomy. Ostomies pouch need to be kept clean. The first step to cleaning and changing the pouch is to collect all the materials required to include: another pouch, pouch clip, towel, scissors, wipes, tissue, card and pen, and stoma powder. Changing can be done when bathing. The pouch can be emptied in a toilet. Then the hands are cleaned, and then the pouch is removed. The clip is retained and the used pouch is thrown to a dustbin wrapped in a plastic bag. Clean the area with clean water using a towel and dry it.

Inspect the skin to see if it is healthy. Use the wipes to clean around the opening and powder the wipes then gently pat the powder to the skin. The skin should be left to dry for two minutes. Measure the stoma then attach the new pouch using the clip. Finally, clean the hands using soap and water (Hampton and Bryant, 1992, p. 4).

14. Emergencies in the home and critical steps to follow.

Emergencies in the home care include clients who are in danger like fire or drowning in water, and sustained injury from a collapse. It can be faint or absence of breathing from client or unconsciousness. Upon recognizing an emergency, the home health aide should move the client from the danger. If they have fallen and have serious injuries, they should avoid moving them. The ambulance can be called right away. The manager in charge of supervising the home health aide should be notified.

15. The chain of infection in the home care setting.

In the home care setting an agent of infection may be found in the hands, equipment, masks or surfaces. The agent of infection will have a reservoir like a surface, equipment, water, air human where they live. They look for an exit through blood and body secretions. The agent of infection is transmitted to another who has contact with the infected (water, food, air or human). The agent gets entry to the body through the nose, digestive organs, reproductive system, respiratory system, skin and circulatory system.

16. Infection control measures to use in the home care setting.

Infections can be controlled in the home setting if hands are cleaned thoroughly very often. The home health aide can take a balanced diet, wash cloths and the body daily. They can get immunized for common infections. Door knobs and other surfaces can be wiped with antiseptic. The mouth can be covered when coughing or sneezing. Waste can be disposed in the trash correctly. The toothbrush can be changed after a few months. Artificial nails can be avoided. It can help for a sick client to stay at home when sick to avoid re-infection and spreading the infection. Moreover, hygiene should be emphasized at all times (Rhinehart and McGoldrick, 2005, 11).

17. Role and responsibilities of the HHA in assisting the client to self-administer medications.

The home health aide role and responsibility in assisting client to self-administer medication includes getting the medicine from the storage and returning after use. Check the labels to confirm the medication is prescribed to the specific client. Observe time and remind the client time for the next dose. Be present as client takes medication and offer help. The client may need juice, spoon and one to open the container. Give support to the hand as the client takes medication, and offer help to return tablets to the container.

18. Conclusion.

Personal care is a significant task in home. Personal care enables the client in home care to be comfortable and prevent infection. Improvised equipment cut down on cost and facilitates homecare delivery. Home care delivery is intended to give the client quality healthcare services. Understanding on body mechanics gives insight on the best way to transfer and move a client. The client needs to exercise for health circulation and muscle strengthening. The skin needs care to prevent it from injuries such as pressure ulcers. The skin can be protected by eating healthy and taking care of it. Infections can be controlled if hygiene is observed.

References

Birchenall, J. M. (2012). Mosby's Textbook for the Home Aide. New Jersey: Mosby.

Birchenall, J. M., and Streight, E. (2003) Mosby's Textbook for the Homecare aide, 2nd edition,   New Jersey: Mosby.

Canadian Pharmacists Association (2002) Patient Self Care, Canada: Canadian Pharmacists.

Cain, B. (1940) Improvised Equipment in the Home Care of the Sick, *American Journal of   Public Health and the Nations Health* 30, 3, 294-294.

Dixon, M. W. (2000) Body Mechanics and Self-Care Manual. New Jersey: Prentice Hall.

Habif, T. P., Campbell, J. L., Chapman, M. S., Dinulos, J. G. H., and Zug, K. A. (2011)Skin Disease: Diagnosis and Treatment, Philadelphia: Saunders.

Hampton, B. and Bryant, R. (1992). Ostomies and Continent Diversions: Nursing Management,
    Missouri: Mosby.

Rhinehart, E., and McGoldrick, M. (2005) Infection Control In Home Care And Hospice,
    Massachusetts: Jones & Bartlett Learning.Shi, L. and Singh, D. A. (2011) Delivering Health Care in

America: A Systems Approach Burlington: Jones &
Bartlett Learning.

Wernig, J. K., and Sorrentine, S. A. (1989).
Homemaker- Home Health Aide. *Journal of Health
Occupation and Education*, 5, 1, 81-82.

CHAPTER FOUR

Nutrition in Home Care

Outline

1. Introduction

2. Key principles of nutrition

3. Potential nutritional problems

4. Therapeutic diets

5. Safe food handling and storage

6. Adaptations for feeding

7. Fluid balancing

8. Community resources for meeting nutritional needs

9. Conclusion

Nutrition in home care.

1. Introduction.

A home care client is depended on good nutrition in their meals if they are to gain energy and strength and restore health. Good nutrition is known to improve the physical body, add to healing and positively contribute to the management of health. This essay will discuss principles of nutrition, give potential problems for lack of nutrition and talk about therapeutic diet. It will highlight safety in handling food, discuss fluid balance and talk about community resources on nutrition.

2. Key principle of nutrition.

According to Gibson (2005, p. 25), adhering to principles of nutrition gives the client strength and helps to maintain body weight. It replaces lost minerals and vitamins, boosts the immune and enhances response after treatment. The client should eat a variety of foods from the following groups; carbohydrates, protein, minerals, fats, vitamins and sugars. The foods should be taken in correct amount to maintain weight and should avoid dehydration by drinking plenty of fluids. The client can have regular exercise. Three main meals in a day with plenty of snacks in between can be adopted.

Ingram and Lavery (2009, p. 218) note that, the body is composed of water, minerals, protein, fats, carbohydrates and refuse. Food that is taken builds the body. Food is important in giving the body energy, warmth and retaining heat and energy.

Implementing nutritional principles enable a person to have energy, good health, and reduce sickness. Eat plenty of fruits and vegetables for good health. Increase water intake. Take seasonal foods since they enhance nutrition. Take a wide variety of diverse foods and ensure food is taken in moderation. Whole food nutrition is better than separate nutrition element. Taking supplements is not an equivalent to replacing food. Take food that is good for eating and not poisonous or contaminated. It is important to discipline self to eat food in the right amount. Good nutrition can prevent and at times reverse illnesses. If nutritional principles are followed the cost of care is reduced since ailments subside.

3. Potential nutrition problems.

Birchenall and Streight (2012, p. 19) mention that, home healthcare clients can experience nutritional problems despite paying attention to getting adequate food. One of the common problems is under nutrition which leads to weight loss. Weight loss can be easily identified and treated with balanced diet, correct food and beverage quantities. However, medication effects and depression that a client experience can lead to weight loss. The problem is solved by introducing feeding tubes to avoid under nutrition of protein energy.

Another problem is deficiency of pyridoxine, folate, vitamin D and minerals like zinc. The deficiency of nutrients hinders healing of wounds and contributes to low immune. Additionally, failure to take adequate fluids causes dehydration. Furthermore, post prandial hypotension can occur and inevitably cause the home care client to have aspiration pneumonia. Aspiration pneumonia can cause a fall.

4. Therapeutic diets.

Therapeutic diets refer to foods that are modified to meet the specific health and physical needs of a client. The modification is recommended by a nutritionist or a medical professional. The objective is to adjust the content of calories, texture or nutrients to the most appropriate depending on the client's condition (William and Schlenker, 2003, p. 17). Therapeutic diets require patience and convincing to the client. This is because they may have body weakness, sickness, lack of appetite or self pity. It is easier to make them understand the use of diet by explanation. Therapeutic diet include food low in cholesterol, food low in residue, regular food, liquid food, soft food, low fat food, food without sodium, food for diabetic and protein diet.

Food low in cholesterol is recommended for clients with heart disease and atherosclerosis. Avoid beef, egg yolk, cheese or food saturated with fats. Food low in residue is best for clients with diarrhea or digestion problems. Regular food can be given to clients with ambulatory needs. Their food should have cream sauce, rich desert, fried foods or salad dressing.

Liquid food is a short term solution for clients recovering from heart attack, surgery and digestion issues. They replace water lost in diarrhea. Soft food is meant for clients who chew little and who have undergone recent surgery. For easy digestion, spicy foods, fried foods, raw fruits and vegetables, coconut, meat or food with tough tissue should be avoided.

Patients with diabetes mellitus have inadequate insulin and should have certain nutrients according to their specific requirements. They should avoid foods or items rich in sugar. Some patients need food high in calorie, while others need food low in calorie. Client with cardiovascular disease should take a low sodium diet. High protein foods are given to children, pregnant mothers, lactating mothers, adolescents and clients after burns or infections. Low protein diet is given to clients with allergic kidney disease as William and Schlenker (2003, p. 17) discuss.

5.   Safe food handling and storage.

The way food is handled, prepared and stored could cause contamination and lead to sickness. Food can be a reservoir that can transmit bacteria from one person to another. Food poisoning can be avoided by preparing and storing food in a clean, safe environment using clean water. Safety can be achieved by observing hygiene. Use clean water for cooking, cleaning and drinking. Clean hands before and after eating food. Contaminated water and food is spread by people, pests and pets.

Another safety principle in food handling is separating raw food from cooked food. In addition food should be cooked for the recommended period using the correct temperature to kill germs. Food should be kept away from contamination and at the recommended temperature. Avoid contaminating safe water or cooked food by keeping it covered (William and Schlenker 2003, p. 19).

6. Adaptations for feeding.

Clients need help to feed. The home health aide will be required to feed the client with healthy and appropriate diet. Home health aide should practice patience and avoid rushing the client to take food. Give attention and focus on feeding the client. Feeding time can be used for conversation. They should show interest and think about client. In case the client is able to feed they should be given independence to feed and get support on arms. The client can be allowed to decide on drinks and foods they prefer to feed on.

The client can be allowed to rest as much as possible and get breaks in between meals. Their food may need to be cooked in a manner that does not make them loose appetite or vomit. It is important to be aware of the bladder and bowel movements, to assess if they need more liquids and fiber. Feed the patients according to their nutritional needs and vary the foods widely. Adjust the nutrition as required from time to time and engage the client as much as possible in the decision making when feeding them.

The client may not be able feed orally and this may cause the patient to use enteral feeding. Enteral feeding is commonly known as tube feeding. Tube feeding is given to patients after a surgery or very ill patients. Tube feeding is safe and allows the caregivers to give nutritional supplements. The feeding tubes have different thickness and are inserted differently according to the individual needs of the client. They require monitoring and accuracy in use to ensure the client is comfortable as they benefit from the feeding. Besides using the feeding tubes as an adaptation for giving nutrition, the feeding tubes can be used to give medication (Bradnam and White, 2010, p. 3).

7. Fluid balancing.

Fluid balance entails ensuring the correct amount of fluid is retained in the body. The input and output should be in continuation. Diseases or illness can be a cause of imbalance and this should be considered when handling specific client's needs. Metheny (2010, p. 9) points out that, reduction of body fluid could cause thirst, illness and sometimes death. Fluid in the body changes with the age, body fat and gender. Fluid is lost with exercise, urination, sweating, hemorrhage, vomiting, diarrhea and diuretics. Fluid is retained if client has liver cirrhosis, has high sodium in the body, and has renal failure, if intravenous fluid is given excessively and where there is congestive cardiac.

Fluid balance assists the body in controlling fluid input and output. As a result, fluid balance ensures there is a

98

balance of the hormones. The home health aide may keep the record of weight, blood pressure, respiration, pulse, urine output, tongue saliva, skin thirst, face and temperature in the management of fluid balance. Therefore fluid balance prevents dehydration, and can restore health after fluid loss following an illness. When the fluid balance record is kept, the information can be used to detect deteriorating health. The client becomes comfortable. Thirst or dryness of tongue, sunken eyes and weakness is uncomfortable. Lack of fluid could cause constipation. Furthermore, fluid imbalance could lead to loss of weight. Fluid balance is necessary because the client may be unable to tolerate deprivation from fluid.

8. Community resources for meeting nutritional needs.

There are programs as well as services offered in the community to assist the sick, elderly, children and those in need to get food services. The services aim at meeting the nutritional needs of specific groups like the children and elderly. The Food and Nutrition Service in United States is one of the agencies that help distribute excess food from farms to the needy. The National School Lunch Program and School Breakfast help meet dietary needs of the school going children. Food Stamp Program educates the low income earners on nutrition and gives stamps to the special groups to access food. The Commodity Supplementary Food Program, Nutrition Program for older America, and Head Start Program allows the elderly to get food, education and transport. The programs and services enable the different groups meet their nutritional needs. There are also community programs that offer home delivered meals, social services and home care services from volunteers.

9. Conclusion.

Nutrition in home care contributes to the health of the client. Principles of nutrition require that protein, carbohydrates, minerals, vitamins, sugars and fats be included in a diet. Food should be taken in correct amount and cooked according to recommended time. Adequate water should be taken and regular exercise adapted. Safe and clean food free from contamination or poison should be avoided. If nutrition is not taken as required the client can lose weight, become dehydrated, get ill, get post prandial hypotension or get aspiration pneumonia. Therapeutic food include: liquid food, regular food, food low in cholesterol, food low in residue, low fat food, food for diabetic, food without sodium, soft food, and protein diet. Food and water should be stored away from contamination. Different clients will need assistance in diet to be able to get nutrition and medication by adapting to diverse texture and method of feeding. Fluids need to be monitored to avoid dehydration or over hydration in the body. The client can get assistance from different services and programs in the community to meet nutritional needs.

Bibliography

Birchenall, J. and Streight, E. (2012) Mosby's Text book for the Home Care Aide. Missouri: Mosby.

Bradnam, V. and White, R.(2010) Handbook of Drug Administration Via Enteral Feeding Tubes,   Illinois: Pharmaceutical Press.

Gibson,   R.   S.   (2005)   Principles   of   nutritional Assessment. USA: Oxford University Press.

Ingram, P. and   Lavery, I. (2009) Clinical skills for healthcare Assistants. John Wiley and Sons.

Metheny, N. M. (2010) Fluid and Electrolyte Balance: Nursing Considerations, Massachusetts: Jones & Bartlett Learning.

William, R. and Schlenker, E. D. (2003) Essentials of Nutrition and Diet Therapy. Mosby.

CHAPTER FIVE

Cleaning tasks in home care

Outline

1. Introduction

2. Role of home health aide

3. Principles of safe home environment

4. Procedure, equipment and supplies for house hold tasks

5. Washing and drying dishes

6. Laundering household and personal items

7. Organizing house hold tasks

8. Conclusion

Cleaning tasks in home care

1. Introduction.

Home care entails maintaining cleanliness and safety in the home. A clean home prevents accumulation of dirt which could be a health hazard and reduces chances of getting infection. This essay describes the role of home health aide in maintaining a clean, safe and healthy environment. The essay further talks about principles of safe home environment and procedures for house hold tasks. It explains how to clean utensils, linen and personal items. Guidelines on organizing the household tasks are discussed in this paper.

2. Role of home health aide.

Home health aide gives safety, cleanliness and health assistance by giving personalized care, checking for physical dangers and report to medical authority about the client. By helping in bathing, dressing and toileting they reduce the chances of discomfort and infections (Prieto, 2008, p. 184).

Assistance in movement, taking medication and feeding reduces accidents. Purchasing, preparing, serving and feeding ensure the client remain healthy. In some cases the home health aide educates the client and family which facilitate their cooperation when it comes to maintaining a safe, clean and healthy environment. Home health aide gives support to client and family by ensuring the surrounding is comfortable and can allow safe mobility (Anene 2009, p. 46).

3. Principles of safe home environment.

To maintain a safe home environment avoid objects that could cause stumbling. One can put hand rails or bars in the house for support. Cabinets with dangerous substances and tools should be locked. Allow temperature for water heater to be adjusted to prevent burns. Naked flames should not be left unattended. Moreover, ensure there is an equipped first aid kit and functional fire extinguisher ready and accessible. Communication should be encouraged.

A safe environment will ensure that there is no risk of burns, drowning, chocking, cuts, falls, loud noise, falling objects, broken items, robes and naked electric wires. It may be necessary to implement a system of monitoring movement like a door alarm, bell or supervision. Ensure there is a working telephone in case of an emergency. The home health aide can practice appropriate body mechanics when moving, lifting and transferring client (Birchenall and Streight 2003, p. 4).

In addition cover the mouth when coughing and wear a mask if the client is coughing frequently. Avoid sitting or standing too close to the patient when they cough or have flu. Ensure there is ventilation to allow flow of fresh air. Soiled cloths, linen and items should be kept away from the clean ones. They can be kept together in a room. The soiled linen can be wrapped so that the soiling is at the middle and does not spill.

4. **Procedure, equipment and supplies for house hold tasks.**

Leahy et al (2008, p. 17) point out that, it is necessary to collect and get the right equipment and supplies to protect self and to avoid infection when cleaning. House hold equipment and supplies required include: broom, mop, dust pan, disinfectant, bleach, rag, scrub brush, vacuum and scrap. Infection control measures should be considered in every procedure. Wear gloves when performing tasks and handling soiled linen, equipment or cloths. Clean hands regularly, preferably before and after completing tasks. Separate dirty and clean areas. The bathroom should be cleaned with cloth and the toilet wiped with a disposable cloth.

When cleaning the kitchen start with the top to bottom, wipe spills and throw garbage daily. To clean the bathroom cleaning starts from top to bottom then clean sinks, shower and then the toilet. The floor and the water spills should be cleaned last. To clean the living room, begin with vacuuming the carpet. If there is no vacuum cleaner, sweep the carpet with a brush, collect garbage and throw it in a dustbin. Loose rags can then be tacked. Dust and wipe the furniture or items and return them to original place. To clean the floor, sweep first, then mop and finally dry the floor.

5. **Washing and drying dishes.**

When washing and drying utensils, it is important to establish if there is any utensils that need sterilization. Those that need regular cleaning should be kept together. To begin the cleaning processes gather all the utensils and equipment for sterilization. Get plenty of water, soft cloth and soap. Sort the utensils according to type and dirt. Clean hands and wash less dirty items first. Wash one item at a time. Avoid overcrowding the utensil because it can cause glass to fall and break. Clean utensils in warm soapy water using a soft dish cloth. Rinse the utensils in clean water, place them in a utensil drying rack and leave them to drip dry for a while. Wipe with a clean dry cloth and place in appropriate place.

If the utensils were to be sterilized clean and place them in a clean pot with cold water. Place the glass at the bottom and avoid overcrowding. Close the top and heat until there is steam. Let the steam sterilize for the next twenty minutes. When the heat is put out and the steam is no longer there open the lid. The lid should be open only if the steam has dispersed. Remove utensils using tongs. Keep the sterilized equipment away from the other utensils that are unsterilized (Rice 2006, p. 85).

6. Laundering household and personal items.

Rice (2006, p. 89) indicates that when laundering household and personal items for a client, wear gloves before beginning the tasks. Sort the soiled and unsoiled cloths and linen first. Get information if the cloths or linen are to be washed using a machine and get the instructions on how to operate it. If they are to be hand washed, it may be necessary to consider wearing gloves and using the disinfectant. Empty any contents that may be found in the pockets. Then sort the cloths and the linen according to color. Some cloths and linen can be cleaned separately if soiled or delicate. Then find out about drying; if to be air dried or to be dried using the drying machine.

7. Organizing house hold tasks.

Household tasks can become overwhelming if proper planning is not done. Begin with a list of household tasks. Then the tasks can be sorted and arranged according to time. Activities can be grouped into daily, weekly and monthly tasks. For example, vacuuming can be done weekly, paying telephone, water and electricity bill monthly, and buying medication upon advice. The rooms can be cleaned once a week. After arranging according to time remove and reduce the unnecessary tasks. For instance, the dishes need more time for cleaning than the fan. Some duties can be designated. If the tasks are too many to handle, one can ask for assistance. This will ensure that all prioritized and necessary tasks are completed. Practice what is in the plan and make adjustments where necessary. When a routine is maintained and adapted household tasks can be accomplished (Gingerch 2008, p. 163).

8. Conclusion.

To create safe, clean and healthy environment, the home health aide practices personalized care and hygiene in giving care. They use body mechanic skills to move patients and educate family together with the client for them to assist in the cooperation of maintaining a clean, safe and healthy environment. Cleanliness is maintained for comfort. Assistance is given in feeding and medication. A safe environment is maintaining by eliminating any danger. The home is cleaned using bleach, a broom, dust pan, scrap, mop, disinfectant, vacuum, and rag and scrub brush. Utensils are washed and dried or disinfected. Lined and personal items are sorted so that the soiled ones are cleaned separately. To organize household tasks, a list of all work is written. The tasks are arranged according to time and the less necessary tasks omitted. Help when there is a lot of work is needed. The plan is followed and adjusted accordingly.

Bibliography

Anene, E. C. (2009) Home Health Aide Training Manual And Handbook, Bloomington: iUniverse.

Birchenall, J. and Streight, E. (2003) Mosby's Text book for the Home Care Aide. Missouri: Mosby.

Gingerich, B. S. (2008) Pocket Guide for the Home Care Aide, Burlington: Jones & Bartlett   Publishers.

Leahy, W., Fuzy, J., and Grefe, J. (2008) Providing Home Care: A Textbook for Home Health   Aides,   3rd Edition. New Mexico: Hartman Publishing, Inc.

Prieto, E. (2008) Home Health Care Provider: A Guide to Essential Skills, New York: Springer   Publishing Company

Rice, R. (2006) Home Care Nursing Practice: Concepts And Application New Jersey: Mosby.

SAMPLE HOME HEALTH AIDE TEST QUESTIONS

51) All human beings have the same basic physical needs which include:

 A) Food and water

 B) Activity

 C) Sleep and rest

 D) All of the above

52) One of the following is not a psychosocial need:

 A) Love and affection

 B) Shelter

 C) Security

 D) Self esteem

53) A system of learned behaviors, practiced by a group of people that are considered to be the tradition of that people is called:

 A) Actualization

 B) Tribe

 C) Culture

 D) Precision

54) ....is the name for the condition in which all of the body's systems are their best?

 A) Homeostasis

 B) Metabolism

 C) Peristalsis

 D) Arthritis

55) Which of the following is not a system of the body?

 A) Endocrine system

B) Diving system

C) Urinary system

D) Nervous system

56) When the outside temperature is too high, the blood vessels:

A) Constrict

B) Becomes excited

C) Dilate

D) Shortens

57) Which of the following gives the body shape and structure?

A) Apocrine and eccrine structures

B) Veins

C) Arteries

D) Bones and ligaments

58) The nervous system controls and coordinates all body functions.

A) True

B) False

59) The taking-in (breathing in) of oxygen by the body is referred to as:

A) Inspiration

B) Expiration

C) Purification

D) Exchange

60) The largest system organ and the system in the body are the:

A) Mouth

B) Skin

C) Esophagus

D) The small intestine

61) One of the following is a common musculoskeletal system disorder?

A) Nephrotic syndrome

B) Histoplasmosis

C) Pneumonia

D) Osteoporosis

62) The digestive system is also called:

A) Respiratory system

B) Gastro-intestinal Tract

C) Metabolic system

D) Nervous system

63) The two major functions of gastrointestinal system are:

A) Digestion and elimination

B) Digestion and locomotion

C) Elimination and respiration

D) None of the above

64) Endocrine glands secrete:

A) Hormones

B) Enzymes

C) Lipase

D) Amylase

65) The sex cells are formed in the male and female sex glands called the:

A) Gonads

B) Androgens

C) Estrogens

D) Lymphatic

66) At age 1-3 toddlers learn to:

A) Choose education

B) Speak

C) Prepare for retirement

D) Develop language skills and vocabularies

67) ....is a disease or condition that will eventually cause death?

A) A recuperating disease

B) An acute condition

C) Reproductive system

D) A terminal disease

68) The term for the special care a dying person needs is called?

A) Skin care

B) Hospice care

C) Recuperation

D) Advancement stage

69) Which of the following is not included in the normal changes of aging?

A) Incontinence

B) Immunity weakens

C) Appetite decreases

D) Short-term memory loss occurs

70) Common disorders found in infancy period include:

A) Prematurity

B) Low birth weight

C) Sudden infant death syndrome

D) All of the above

71) Which of the following are the basic body positions?

A) Supine

B) Lateral

C) Prone

D) All of the above

72) One of the most important things to consider when transferring a client to a chair or a bed is:

A) Safety

B) Nutrition

C) The Family

D) Finance

73) Contractures are generally caused by:

A) Exercise

B) Driving

C) Locomotion

D) Immobility

74) Pulling a client across sheets can cause:

A) Fluid retention

B) Shearing

C) Spinal cord damage

D) None of the above

75) …………..is a device, such as splint or a brace, which helps support and align a limb and improve its functioning?

A) Leaning table

B) An orthotic device

C) Hand role

D) Head pillows

76) Hygiene and grooming activities, as well as dressing, eating and toileting are called?

A) Activities of daily living

B) Recreational activities

C) Indoor activities

D) Unhealthy life styles

77) Oral care should be performed at least:

A) Once a day

B) At bed time

C) Twice a day

D) None of the above

78) …………….is the inhalation of food, fluid or foreign material into the lungs?

A) Expiration

B) Inspiration

C) Aspiration

D) Asphyxia

79) Moving a body part towards the midline of the body is referred to as:

A) Supination

B) Phonation

C) Rotation

D) Adduction

80) One of the following is not done if a client starts to fall during a transfer?

A) Try to reverse or stop a fall

B) Widen your stance

C) Call for help if a family member is around

D) Do not try to reverse or stop a fall

81)................is the impairment of physical or mental functions:

A) A disability

B) Burn

C) Neuralgia

D) Heart failure

82) A fallacy is:

A) An opinion

B) Truth

C) Being sure

D) A false belief

83) Which of the following can cause mental illness or make it worse?

A) Heredity

B) Stress

C) Environmental factors

D) All of the above

84) Sadness is the only one symptom of:

A) Happiness

B) Depression

C) Hopefulness

D) Excitement

85) Arthritis causes:

A) Dementia

B) Tuberculosis

C) Constipation

D) Stiffness and pain

86) In diabetes mellitus, the pancreas does not produce enough:

A) Estrogen

B) Prolactin

C) Insulin

D) Progesterone

87) Type 2 diabetes can also be referred to as:

A) Adult-onset diabetes

B) Electrically-charged insufficiency

C) Childbearing diabetes

D) All of the above

88) Paralysis on one side of the body is called:

A) Hemiplegia

B) Aphasia

C) Quadriplegia

D) Dysphagia

89) Risk factors for cancer include the following, except:

A) Poor nutrition

B) Water

C) Radiation

D) Tobacco use

90) A brain disorder that affects a person's ability to think and communicate clearly is called:

A) Anemia

B) AIDS

C) Paresis

D) Schizophrenia

91) Which of the following practices are accepted during housekeeping?

A) Be organized when performing tasks

B) Main a safe environment

C) Familiarize yourself with the household's cleaning materials

D) All of the above

92) Cleaning of the kitchen should be done:

A) Once a day

B) At night only

C) After every use

D) Once in a week

93) Which of the following is an example of a detergent?

A) Soap

B) Iodine

C) Kerosene

D) Anion

94) The process of giving special treatment to items that have heavy soil, spots,, and stains before washing them is called:

A) Retreating

B) Escalation

C) Retouching

D) Pretreating

95) Which of the following would be the reason for changing bed linens?

A) The sheets are wrinkled, making a client uncomfortable

B) The linen was used by another client

C) The linen is damp or unclean

D) All of the above

96) The process by which nutrients are broken down to be used by the body for energy and other needs is referred to as:

A) Reproduction

B) Metabolism

C) Excitation

D) Lyses

97) There are ………….nutrients needed by the body for growth and development:

A) Three

B) Two

C) Six

D) Four

98) Foods high in sodium include the following, except:

    A) Bacon

    B) Ham

    C) Sausage

    D) Orange

99) The state of being frightened, excited, confused, in danger or irritated is referred to as:

    A) Stress

    B) Joy

    C) Mood change

    D) None of the above

100)…………..occurs when a person does not have enough fluid in his body?

    A) Dehydration

    B) Fluid overload

    C) Crackles in the lungs

    D) Water toxicity

CHAPTER SIX

Prevention of Infection in Home Health Care

Outline

Introduction

Types of infections encountered in home care

Modes of transmission and ways of prevention

Personal Protective Equipment (PPE) in home   health

care

Conclusion

Introduction

Although the level and extent to which infection acquired at a hospital during treatment has been exhaustively discussed, measured, and analyzed within a litany of different medical research journals and studies, the level to which infectious disease exists within the home treatment realm is an issue that has received a far reduced level of focus. This of course is due to the fact that a far smaller percentage of individuals receive home care; however, due to the fact that it represents a growing percentage of the means of health care delivery, the question itself has significance within the context of nursing and medicine. As such, this brief analysis will seek to analyze the definition of infection, types of infection/most common types of infection that exist within home health care, the modes of these different infection transmissions, ways to impede or disrupt such transmissions, and self-protective equipment and its application within the home health care setting.

Though home health care accounts for but a small percentage of total health care delivery within the United States, it is nonetheless a growing sector of health care deserves discussion. According to a recent study, published in 2011, there has been a high level of growth within home care; however, it still pales in comparison to the total amount

124

of money that is expended upon hospital care. As of 2011, home care represented just 3% of total health care expenditures as compared to over 31% of total expenditure taking place with relation to traditional hospitals. However, the fact remains that even though the figure is small; it is a growing sector and is expected to grow a further 2.5% in the coming decade. As such, it is necessary to understand some of the key nuances that exist within home care as a function of anticipating and treating these issues in a medically expeditious means.

For purposes of this brief analysis, the author will consider infection to be, "the invasion of a host organism's bodily tissues by disease-causing organisms, their multiplication, and the reaction of the host tissues to these organisms and the toxins they produce" (Krismer 2012). With such a broad and encompassing definition, it becomes clear that infection within home care encompasses a broad range of issues; some acting as a more primal threat to health than others. It is important to note that although many journal entries have warned concerning the level of latent disease and exposure that exists within hospital and primary care, the level to which pathogens exist within the environment of the home is far less uniform. Whereas hospitals most comply with federal standards of cleanliness and procedures for disposal of an array of disease causing agents, regularly schedule cleanings, and a host of other preventative mechanisms, home care is almost invariably not nearly so tightly regulated, or sanitary. For this very reason, the prevalence of disease and the severity with which it affects patients within the given context is almost invariably higher than a similarly community of patients within a traditional medical facility. However, the prevalence of infection within the home care theater is not reason in and of itself to strongly recommend against its implementation as a means of treatment.

Types of infections encountered in home care

With regards to the types of infections and the most common infections that exhibit themselves within home care, there are a number which will herein be discussed. As one might expect, the very same infectious disease agents that exhibit themselves within the hospital care front are also exhibited within home care; albeit, to different extents and total percentage rates than in traditional hospital care. For instance, studies on home care have typically indicated that the most common types of infections are concentric upon urinary tract infections, followed by an array of different types of skin infections, with staphylococcus aureus, and enterococcus rounding out the least likely but still statistically significant forms of infection exhibited in home care (Patte et al 2009). The presentation of these particular infections is useful to note due to the face that approximately 6% of the home care patients that have been sampled in different studies have reported infection rates that reflect the aforementioned issues. As a means of understanding the overall prevalence and signs of these diseases, the health care professional can attempt to recognize key symptoms as well as make the steps necessary to ensure that aggravating factors do not contribute to a worsening of the patient's condition.

Modes of Transmission and ways of prevention

As with any form of infection, the means of transmission can almost always be attributed to contact in one shape or form with a contaminated object or organism. In this sense, the previously discussed information concerning the difficulty in seeking to sterilize the home environment as compared to that of the hospital is brought to mind. Although individuals would often like to think of their home as a superior place with respect to overall cleanliness and presence of disease as compared to that of a hospital, such is not the case. Moreover, the fact of the matter is that the different disease carrying agents that exist within the home provide for a veritable Petri dish of infectious agents which could negatively impact the health of the patient. Additionally, although the patient or caregivers of the patients may seek to invoke the logic that the "pathogens" that exist within the home are somehow harmless and the patient has been exposed to them their entire life, the inevitable truth is that the patient is in a highly weakened state and likely has never spent time at the home before at a time in which their immune system and overall health are at such a precarious state (Managan et al 2003). For this reason alone, it is necessary to place a high level of emphasis on seeking to both counteract and prepare for the eventualities that the home care avenue of patient care will necessarily present key challenges that the healthcare professional must differentiate from that of the traditional healthcare model; as exhibited by care within a primary care facility.

Lastly, seeking to ameliorate the risk of transmission for the pathogens that have thus far been discussed within the arena of home care, the practitioner should seek to both employ the same practices that help to ensure that infectious pathogens are kept at a minimum within the hospitals as well as seeking to impart as much knowledge and best practices as possible to the shareholders within the home. In such a manner, activities that would otherwise spread germs and provide a level of threat to the patient in home care must be sought to be identified as well as reduced or discontinued entirely (Rinehart 2001). Rather than merely pointing out one or two areas in which the spread of key types of pathogens could be reduced, such an approach requires that the healthcare professional be mindful and highly attuned to the individual nature of the household's that the patient is receiving home care within. In such a way, the healthcare professional will be able to offer insightful advice and guidance with respect to providing as sanitary and pathogen-free a zone of care as is possible. An example is if the home health aide notices that plates are not washed on time, or that dirty linens are reused over and over, pointing this out to the family as a method of harboring infection is very vital. Another simple example is not using gloves when changing diapers.

Personal protective equipment in home health care

In the same way, many of the same tools that are utilized within the hospital can also be utilized within the arena of home care. For instance, proper use of gloves, masks, and other pathogen reduction means can be utilized as a means of protecting the patient from pathogens born both within the house and from the outside environment into the home (Weber et al 2009). Although advanced hospital practices such as sterilization of equipment and tools cannot take place within the home, the ability to utilize the aforementioned means as a way to minimize the threat of disease is not insignificant.

Conclusion

Although health care within the home environment exhibits a level of key concerns and dangers that traditional hospital care does not necessarily espouse, the considerations proposed within this chapter help the reader to understand some of the means by which the threats of infection can be lessened through the proper application of key knowledge. As a means of seeking to continually providing a higher level of care, while at the same time providing the end-consumer with the means by which they can take a level of self-determination within the realm of healthcare, it is doubtless that the utilization and application of home care will only continue to grow and expand within the coming years. As such, seeking to understand the key ways in which the medical community can work to sanitize the environment as well as educate the key healthcare shareholders in the process has a direct effect on the overall efficacy of the process.

References

Krismer, M. (2012). Definition of infection. *Hip International*, S2-S4. doi:10.5301/HIP.2012.9563

Manangan, L. P., Pearson, M. L., Tokars, J. I., Miller, E., & Jarvis, W. R. (2003). National Surveillance of Healthcare-Associated Infections in Home Care Settings -- Feasible or Not?. *Journal Of Community Health Nursing, 20*(4), 223-231.

Patte, R., Drouvot, V., Quenon, J., Denic, L., Briand, V., & Patris, S. (2005). Prevalence of hospital-acquired infections in a home care setting. *Journal Of Hospital Infection, 59*(2), 148-151.

Rhinehart, E. (2001). Infection Control in Home Care. *Emerging Infectious Diseases, 7*(2), 208.

Weber, D., Brown, V., Huslage, K., Sickbert-Bennett, E., & Rutala, W. (2009). Device-related infections in home health care and hospice: infection rates, 1998-2008. *Infection Control & Hospital Epidemiology, 30*(10), 1022-1024. doi:http://dx.doi.org/10.1086/605641

Chapter 7

Vital Signs

Vital signs can reflect the functions of three body processes necessary for life:

Body temperature

Respiration

Heart function

The four vital signs of body function are:

Temperature

Pulse

Respiration

Blood pressure

Temperature

Body temperature is a balance between heat production and heat loss in conjunction with each other, maintained and regulated by the hypothalamus.

Thermometers are used to measure temperature using the Fahrenheit and Centigrade or Celsius scale. Temperature sites are the following: mouth, rectum, ear (tympanic membrane), and the axilla (underarm). The normal ranges for each site are:

Site	Normal Range
Rectal	98.6Fto 100.6F (37.0C to 38.1C)
Oral	97.6F to 99.6F (36.5C to 37.5C)
Axillary	96.6F to 98.6F (35.9C to 37.0C)
Tympanic Membrane	98.6F (37C)

Some terms used to describe body temperature are:

Febrile – presence of fever

Afebrile – absence of fever

Fever – elevated body temperature beyond normal range. Types of fever are:

Intermittent: fluctuating fever that returns to or below baseline then rises again.

Remittent: fluctuating fever that remains elevated; it does not return to baseline

temperature.

Continuous: a fever that remains constant above the baseline; it does not fluctuate.

Oral temperature is the most common method of measurement; however, it is not taken

from the following patients:

- infants and children less than six years old
- patients who has had surgery or facial, neck, nose, or mouth injury
- those receiving oxygen
- those with nasogastric tubes
- patients with convulsive seizure
- hemiplegic patients
- patients with altered mental status

Wait for 30 minutes to take the oral temperature in patients who have just finished eating, drinking, or smoking. When taking the temperature, leave the thermometer in the patient's mouth for 3-5 minutes or as required by agency policy.

Rectal temperature is taken when oral temperature is not feasible. However, it is not taken from the following patients:

- patients with heart disease
- patients with rectal disease or disorder or has had rectal surgery
- patients with diarrhea

It is taken with the patient in a side-lying position and the thermometer and the patient's hip is held throughout the procedure so the thermometer is not lost in the rectum or broken.

Axillary temperature is the least accurate and is taken only when no other temperature site can be used. The axilla, (the underarm) should be clean and dry and the thermometer should be held in place for 5-10 minutes or as required by the facility policy.

Tympanic temperature is useful for children and confused patients because of the speed of operation of the tympanic thermometer. A covered probe is gently inserted into the ear canal and temperature is measured within seconds (1–3 seconds). It is not used if the patient has an ear disorder or ear drainage.

Pulse

The normal adult pulse rate ranges between 60 and 100 beats per minute. The site most
commonly used for taking pulse is the radial artery found in the wrist on the same side as the thumb. It is felt with the first two or three fingers (never with the thumb) and usually taken for 30 seconds multiplied by two to get the rate per minute. If the rate is unusually fast or slow, however, count it for 60 seconds.

The apical pulse is a more accurate measurement of the heart rate and it is taken over the apex of the heart by auscultation using the stethoscope. It is used for patients with irregular heart rate and for infants and small children.

Respiration

When measuring respiration, respiratory characteristics such as rate, rhythm, and depth are taken into account. Rate is the number of respirations per minute. The normal range for adults is 12 to 20 per minute. One inspiration (inhale) and one expiration (exhale) counts as one respiration. It is counted for 30 seconds multiplied by two or for a full minute.

Some rate abnormalities are the following:

Apnea – this is a temporary complete absence of breathing which may be a result of a

reduction in the stimuli to the respiratory centers of the brain.

Tachypnea – this is a respiration rate of greater than 40/min. It is transient in the newborn and maybe caused by the hysteria in the adult.

Bradypnea – decrease in numbers of respirations. This occurs during sleep. It may also

be due to certain diseases.

Respiratory rhythm refers to the pattern of breathing. It can vary with age: infants have an irregular rhythm while adults have regular.

Some abnormalities in the rhythm are the following:

Cheyne-Stokes – this is a regular pattern of irregular breathing rate.

Orthopnea – this is difficulty or inability to breath unless in an upright position.

Depth of respiration refers to the amount of air that is inspired and expired during each respiration. Some abnormalities in the depth of respirations are the following:

Hypoventilation: state in which reduced amount of air enters the lungs resulting in

decreased oxygen level and increased carbon dioxide level in blood. It can be due to breathing that is too shallow, or too slow, or to diminished lung function.

Hyperpnea: abnormal increase in the depth and rate of breathing.

Hyperventilation: state in which there is an increased amount of air entering the lungs.

Blood Pressure

This is the measurement of the amount of force exerted by the blood on the peripheral arterial walls and is expressed in millimeters (mm) of mercury (Hg). The measurement consist of two components: the highest (systole) and lowest (diastole) amount of pressure exerted during the cardiac cycle.

A stethoscope and sphygmomanometer of either aneroid or mercury type are used. The size of the cuff of the sphygmomanometer will depend on the circumference of the limb and not the age of the patient. The width of the inflatable bag within the cuff should be about 40% of this circumference – 12 cm to 14 cm in an average adult. The length of the bag should be about 80% of this circumference – almost long enough to encircle the arm. Cuffs that are too short or narrow may give falsely high readings, e.g. a regular cuff on an obese arm may lead to a false diagnosis of hypertension.

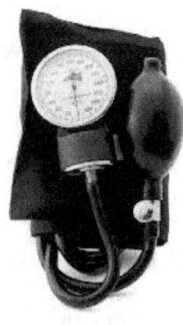

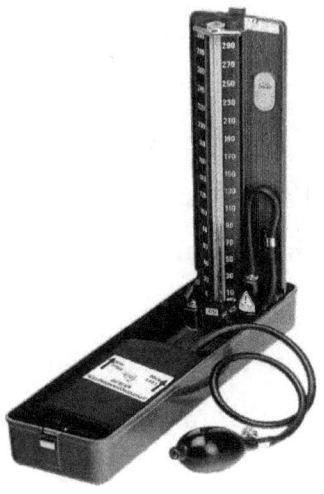

The inflatable bag is centered over the brachial artery with the lower border about 2.5cm above the antecubital crease. The cuff is positioned at heart level. If the brachial artery is far below the heart level the blood pressure will appear falsely high. If the brachial artery is far above heart level, blood pressure will appear falsely low.

Blood pressure is taken by determining first the palpatory systolic pressure over the brachial artery. Then with the bell of the stethoscope over the brachial artery, the cuff is inflated again to about 30 mm Hg above the palpatory systolic pressure and deflated slowly, allowing the pressure to drop at a rate of about 2 to 3 mmHg per second. Note the level at which you hear the sounds of at least two consecutive beats. This is the systolic pressure. Continue to lower the pressure slowly until the sounds become muffled and then disappear. Then deflate the cuff rapidly to zero. The disappearance point, which is usually only a few mmHg below the muffling point, marks the generally accepted diastolic pressure. Both the systolic and diastolic pressure levels are read the nearest 2 mmHg.

Common errors in blood pressure measurements:

Improper cuff size. Cuffs that are too short or narrow may give falsely high readings. Using a regular cuff on an obese arm may lead to a false diagnosis of hypertension. For an obese arm, select a cuff with a larger than standard bag.

The arm is not at heart level. If the brachial artery is much below the heart level, the blood pressure will appear falsely high. Conversely, if the artery is much above heart level, blood pressure will appear falsely low. A 13.6 cm difference between arterial and cardiac levels produces a blood pressure error of 10mmHg.

Cuff is not completely deflated before use. Deflation of the cuff is faster than 2-3 mmHg per second. Rapid deflation will lead to underestimation of the systolic and overestimation of the diastolic

pressure.

The cuff is re-inflated during the procedure without allowing the arm to rest for 1-2 minute between readings. Repetitive inflation of the cuff can result in venous congestion, which could make the sound less audible producing artifactually low systolic and high diastolic pressure.

Improper cuff placement.

Defective equipment. A bag that balloons outside the cuff leads to falsely high readings.

BONUS READING FOR HOME CARE-GIVERS

PART ONE: The Ideal Caregiver

Who is the ideal caregiver?

The ideal caregiver is someone who fulfills all the following roles and qualities:

1. Knows his/her responsibilities
2. Knows his/her limitations
3. Carries out his/her job professionally
4. Maintains personal hygiene
5. Maintains punctuality
6. Maintains his/her own safety
7. Has good observation skills and good initiatives
8. Very open to suggestions
9. Has a sense of humor
10. Takes pride in his/her job

Responsibilities

The responsibilities of the caregiver include but are not limited to the following:

- Routine personal care
- Hygiene assistance
- Laundry
- Cleaning
- Shopping
- Meal planning and cooking

- Rides to doctor appointments and errands
- Medication reminders

Limitations

The caregiver should know that he/she is at this home to care. She/he is not biologically part of this family and as such does not have certain rights. There are times when she may have access to a patient's personal information like bank accounts, social security number, some Identification cards, and other private information. The limitations of her job must always come to his/her mind. These information should not be discussed outside the home of the patient. The information should not, in some cases even be discussed with the patient as he/she may become suspicious and start feeling uncomfortable around her and possibly dismiss her from the job. The caregiver is not to make certain decisions for her patients. When some vital decisions are to be made, the patient's son or daughter or significant other should be called to make the decision.

Professionalism

The free online dictionary defines professionalism as "the expertness characteristic of a professional person";" skillfulness by virtue of possessing special knowledge". [1] From this definition we can simply say that being professional means that one knows the skills of her job and delivers them with expertise. For a caregiver, do not feel intimated that you are serving, be very humble and carry out your responsibilities with expertise. The way you present yourself determines how you are valued and respected before your client. Remember that respect is not demanded but commanded. It is also very imperative that caregivers use appropriate clothing to work. Very tight fitting jeans or pants should be avoided. Revealing tops should also be avoided. The best clothes to wear to a caregiver job are scrubs.

I remember a certain day that a caregiver walked in and the aroma of the environment changed. I thought in my mind "Does it mean that this lady cannot perceive this odor?" I

---

[1] http://www.thefreedictionary.com/professionalism

looked at the faces of those around me and I saw 'that look'. Other people were as uncomfortable as I was but no one dared told her what was happening. It looked like she left her scrubs in the washing machine overnight before drying it. But wait a minute. Couldn't she smell that? I started imagining what would happen when this lady bends over a patient to take care of him/her; that poor patient will definitely not find it funny! Should we maintain personal hygiene as caregivers? The answer is a bold YES! There is no such excuse as "I was late so I forgot to shower" or statements of that sort. Better be late and clean.

Punctuality

According to wordnetweb, punctuality means "the quality or habit of adhering to an appointed time"[2] Caregivers need to adhere to the appointed time for the start of shift. I once interviewed one of my clients, and the old woman commended a caregiver I sent to her "She is always her by 9 am, very punctual!" That made me feel very good as the employer. Sometimes caregivers could meet traffic or things of the sort. In order to maintain punctuality leave

_____

[2] http://wordnetweb.princeton.edu/perl/webwn?s=punctuality

your house earlier than you should to give room for traffic emergencies. The issue at hand is your arrival on time, not the excuses that made you not to.

Maintenance of safety will be treated as a different topic.

Good observation skills and initiatives: Do you know the game 'bingo'? If you have played bingo or knows about it, you will remember that it requires a lot of alertness both in quick observation of the numbers and the ability to shout bingo first. The care giving job is a little like bingo because it demands a lot of observation and alertness. Your patient has been left under your care. Erase it from your mind that she/he can stay without you; have it your mind that as far as you are in that house she is under your care and so deserves your complete attention. Observe for mood changes, signs of hunger, pain, etc. which she may feel uncomfortable to voice out. Ask open ended questions like "I see that your face is not very bright, is there something you want to talk about?" Be very polite and do not push for the patient to give you the information that she does not want to. Initiative means embarking on new ventures. In the case of senior care, I would explain it to mean the ability to think fast of the solution of an immediate problem. An example is this: you find your patient slump all of a sudden while eating at the dining table, what do you do? Many ideas run through your mind like "Run!" "Call the daughter or son" "Call 911" "Call your agency" "Start CPR". All these ideas are very vital and should all be done (except of course,"Run!") but should be placed in the correct order and this is the correct order: "Call 911", "Start CPR" but if you suspect a fracture, stop and don't move the patient. When the emergency team arrives, call the significant other then call your agency. In the case of an emergency as described, be sure to give accurate information to the emergency team. Give as much correct information as you know and only those needed for the care.

Openness to suggestions

The caregiver must be open to suggestions given by her agency and the family. It is always good to remember that you are there to serve.

Has a sense of humor

When I started practicing as a nurse, I would come to work, take my duties so seriously, trying to be the best nurse, do my job and go home. As time went on, I started finding out that my colleagues were not very comfortable with me. Why? I soon found out: I was 'too serious' with my work. It was not until I brought my real funny self and started expressing my sense of humor that everyone started changing their minds about me. There is more to life. Season every second as much as you can. That will make you enjoy your job and feel at home to leave your house the next day. Moreover, that will make your clients want you to always be there for them.

Takes pride in the job

Have you ever seen someone who hates his job? He makes a lot of mistakes at the job, creates a lot of bad impressions, gets depressed on the job and never retains one job for too long. I want to say that the care giving job is a noble profession because it is not everyone that possesses the gift to care for others. So, my dear caregiver, take pride in your job!

"The caregiver needs to feel good about themselves. If you don't feel good, you won't respond well to a difficult situation."

Kathleen O'Brien

More explanations on the ideal caregiver

A caregiver can be anybody who helps a person when he/she is in need of it. In general, people suffering from acute illnesses need the help of caregivers. An ideal care giver is one who in addition to looking after the patients, also helps them with their grocery shopping, house cleaning, cooking, shopping, paying bills, giving medicine, bathing, using the toilet, dressing and eating. Individuals who do not charge a penny when it comes to taking care of patients are referred to as family caregivers or informal caregivers.

If your loved one is suffering from any acute illness, you can be by his/her side to help. Most health centers may need patients to have a caregiver for helping them throughout the treatment. As a caregiver you need to provide emotional support to the patient. In addition to this, you need to also act as his/her advocate. As a caregiver, your prime responsibility lies in playing a viable role in the treatment and recovery of your loved one. You need to learn more about your patient's

/patients' disease as well as treatment options as it will help you to make good choices about your care.

Role of an ideal care giver

As a caregiver, you need to remember that you are an eminent member of the heath care group. You need to play a viable role all through the patient's treatment starting from planning to recovery process.

It is quite obvious on your part to feel thrown into a strange world of test results, treatment choices and medical terms if your loved one is suffering from any acute disease. You may have to gather all possible information on earth about the disease, consult doctors, and stay by your patient's side supporting him/her. In simple words, that's what we call an ideal caregiver.

Each patient's needs are different. For example, a patient suffering from autism will have different needs when compared with a patient suffering from Alzheimer's disease. Hence, as a caregiver you need to find your own way of catering to those needs. Irrespective of the different needs, what is expected from an ideal caregiver is love and support throughout the treatment, recovering or peaceful death procedure.

Taking up the responsibility of being a caregiver may turn out to be an overwhelming job. In fact, it helps if you are aware of your job and responsibilities.

- As a caregiver, your first job involves finding out the expectations of the hospital or rather the doctors from you. Many health centers provide special sessions for helping caregivers learn what they need to do when it comes to taking care of patients. For home caregivers, you need to find out the expectations of the family from you.
- Talk to your patient about what they need. For instance, some patients may need only emotional support from you and leave the task of talking to doctors as your advocate to others. On the flip side, some patients may ask you to take up their complete responsibility starting from grocery shopping, giving medicines to providing emotional aid.

You need to act as your patient's advocate. In other words, you need to act as an active supporter of your patient. You can act as your patient's advocate in a number of spheres such as:

- Medical: Being an active member of the health care group, your job lies in gathering information, talking to the physicians together with taking care of the patient at the time of his/her recovery.
- Financial: If your patient has asked you look after his/her financial matters as well then you may talk to the insurance and manage health costs as well as routine household finances.
- Emotional as well as social: Be by your patient's side and listen to what he/she has to say to you.

You can maintain regular updates about your patients in any way that can only be accessible to you. You can write down the names, maps, phone numbers, questions, instructions, and much in a diary. As a caregiver, you need to see to it that the medical team answers all your queries. If you can't be available when the doctor pays a visit to your patient, you can fix a time according to your convenience for talking about your patient's progress to the doctor. Don't be scared of asking questions regarding the patient's progress till you get a satisfactory answer. There are quite a few things that may take place just as expected. Complications may take place and the recovery period may last for quite a long time than expected. You may come across situation when you need to re-admit your patient no sooner than you have brought him/her home. An ideal care giver is one who plans for setbacks, surprises as well as delays. Try focusing on things that you may manage at present and measure the progress of your patient in small increments.

There is a lot to care giving even after the patient leaves the clinic or hospital. In fact, the real care giving job starts off at this juncture. During the first weeks or months after your patient returns home, things may not be that normal. Being a caregiver, you job involves administering medications, Changing colostomy bags, checking the patient's blood sugar, as well as monitoring the patient for infection as well as other complications. Taking the care of a patient at home is much more challenging as compared to taking the care of a patient when at hospital.

Family members as well as friends may not always understand the hard core truth that difficulties never come to an end after the return of the patient from the hospital. In fact, this is the time when a patient needs maximum support from the care giver.

While dealing with a patient, your prime responsibility lies in maintaining an optimistic outlook and a good sense of humor. It is true that dealing with a patient suffering from acute illness is not a matter of joke, but many caregivers know that by maintaining a good sense of humor, they have helped patients to cope up with their illness.

An ideal care giver adjusts to the needs of the patient

The need of a patient at the time of the diagnosis will certainly differ from his/her need at the time of the recovery procedure. An ideal care giver is one who is familiar with the changing responsibilities well in advance. Over and above, this approach of his will help in carrying out the below mentioned transitions more conveniently:

- Helping your patient in preparing for the treatment

- Care giving at the hospital

- Care giving after the patient returns home

Sharing your care giving responsibilities with others

For caregivers who are part of the family, you may try sharing your care giving role with others. Even if you play the chief role in managing the aforementioned areas, you can always delegate some tasks to others. In fact, if you want to be an ideal caregiver, then you need to take utmost care of your own self as well. Hence, it would be advisable on your part if you assign small tasks to others and use your energy in helping the patient which they need you the most.

Often, an individual acts as the main caregiver of the patient. Despite this fact, at times it becomes difficult to carry out the task single-handedly. To avoid this situation, a group of individuals can work jointly as caregivers. When a group shares the role of care giving, communication and organization are keys to success.

Meeting your own needs as care giver

Many a time, caregivers neglect themselves while taking care of others. This could work out for short-term care giving but in long term care giving, It definitely will lead to problems. Some problems that could occur when caregivers put themselves last include but are not limited to: 1. Their becoming ill, 2. Their hating the job 3. Their becoming depressed. 4. Their not delivering appropriate care to their care recipient and thus suffer both themselves and the care recipients.

One of the problems that caregivers usually face is the problem of time. When someone starts the job of care giving, it will not take long to discover that the extra time that was once available is no longer there. This is a big issue and that is why the solution needs to be discussed. Have you ever wondered why the united states made 3 12-hour shifts the full time job for healthcare professional (for those who run 12-hour shifts)? This is because they want to prevent the burn-out associated with care giving. I cannot count the number of times that I forgot to eat while I was working in the hospital. It will start by my saying "I will eat in 15 minutes" and then 15 minutes turns to 30 and 30 turns to 2 hours and sometimes no food till the end of the shift. I cannot count the number of times I had to run into the pantry just to grab an apple juice because my body needed some food. I did not do this every day but I certainly cannot count how many times I have put myself last. From my inquiries, this is not just MY PROBLEM, it is the problem of many caregivers – putting ourselves last.

In order to prevent the burn-out, frustration and depression that accompanies care giving, it is vital to keep some time during the day for yourself. When I learnt this principle, I would gladly hand over my responsibility to the next person and go for lunch or just for a break. In home care, it will depend on the number of hours required of you, if you are doing a four to six hour job, then you can do without a break. But if it is longer, find time to take care of yourself. I remember a day in the hospital that two nurses were quarrelling because one nurse was almost urinating on her herself while the other was still in the restroom. The question now arose "Why did this nurse wait till the last minute before going to the restroom to urinate" The answer is simple. She put herself last. In home care, find time to go to the restroom when it is safe so that you do not endanger the safety of the one receiving your care. Imagine holding a patient in your hands who is depending on you not to fall and at the same time, you are trying to hold back your urine from dripping on your pants!

Meeting your own requirements is important as well. In other words, if you want to be an ideal caregiver, then you need to stay in good health.

An ideal caregiver is one who in addition to taking care of the patients, takes care of him/her as well. When a person is diagnosed with an acute illness and is struggling in between life and death, people are so engrossed with the patient that they often overlook that most important partner of the patient, i.e. the caregiver.

Caring for a person suffering from an acute illness often turns out to be an emotionally draining as well as physically challenging venture. Watching your loved one passing through strenuous medical procedures may change the mind of the most optimistic and healthiest caregiver. Not only this, some care givers feel that their physical health have declined to a considerable extent over the years due to the physical and emotional strains involved in the care giving job. To avoid these consequences, this book introduces some vital points that would help them in meeting personal needs as care givers.

- Care giving is a responsibility and breaks are your deserved right. Hence be sure to reward your own self with occasional breaks.

- Look out for symptoms of depression and never delay when it comes to seeking professional help. The sooner you got better, the sooner you will be able to take care of your patients.

- If people come forward to share your responsibility as a caregiver, don't hesitate. Instead assign them simple tasks that they can carry out easily. You can assign them some of the daily as well as weekly tasks.

- Talk to your friends or try spending some moments away from the patient. You can utilize this time in doing anything that helps you feel relaxed. Check out something that reminds you about the most pleasurable moments of your life.

- Talk to someone who can provide you emotional support. Friends and family members are of great help at this point of time. They are good listeners with whom you may share your feelings.

Professional counseling, talks with support groups and clergy are also good ways of support.

- Concentrate on the significant tasks, keep your energy reserved for helping your patients with things they need the most.

- You can't be an ideal caregiver if you are sick or exhausted. Hence, try eating well balanced meals, exercise regularly and sleep well. Devote some time for your own self. Whether you go for a movie, a walk or visit your friend place, your prime objective should be to take out some time for yourself.

- Ask your family member or friend to act as your advocate, in the like manner as you act as your patient's advocate. Your advocate may keep an eye on you and provide you with the support as well as the time you crave for.

- Appreciate your own self for your care giving job. At times, people are so busy with the patient that they simply turn a deaf ear towards the effort put forward by the caregiver. At times, even the patient is too tired and sick to reward your efforts.

- Take adequate care of your back as your care giving job may demand too much of pulling, pushing and lifting.

- Have faith in your instincts as they are most likely to show you the right direction.

It has been mentioned earlier that individuals who do not charge a penny when it comes to take care of patients are referred to as family caregivers or informal caregivers. Let us now check out a couple of suggestions to help family caregivers when it comes to taking care of the patients.

- As a caregiver, you need to jot down all your questions in pen and paper so that you don't forget them

- Try being clear when it comes to talking about the patient to the doctor. Don't ramble up things at this juncture

- If there are innumerable concerns that you need to discuss, then try going for a consultation appointment. This approach allows you as well as the physician to discuss the progress of the patient in an unhurried manner.

- Keep your own self updated about the disability or disease of the patient. You can also surf the internet for this purpose.

- Check out the routine at the hospital or doctor's chamber so that you can find a suitable time to discuss about the patient's progress.

- Keep aloof your anger and your sense of helplessness about not being able to help your patient.

- Keep in mind that the doctor will try his level best to recover your patient.

Care givers generally share a close if not too close relationship with their patients. Each caregiver and patient is in no way similar to each other. Sometimes, the viewpoint of a patient is likely to differ from the viewpoint of a care giver. Hence, it would be advisable on your part if you try talking to your patient and in the process to find out what he/she needs at each and every phase of illness.

An ideal care giver is one who adapts his or her service for addressing the needs of the patient. The patient and the caregiver need to discuss their expectations (i.e. what sort of responsibilities they need from each other). If possible, they can also jot down their agreement in pen and paper in the form of an agreement. For being an ideal care giver, you need to know the difference between doing and caring. Welcome ideas as well as technologies that promote the independence of your patient. Try updating your own self about the condition of your patient and make sure to communicate with the doctor in an efficient manner.

Good communication is believed to be the most viable quality of a caregiver. In fact, this quality turns out to be more important when caregiver is an immediate family member. There may be times when the patient feels hesitant to speak about his/her actual health condition simply because he/she feels that by doing so he/she will burden the care giver.

An ideal caregiver is one who is an expert in time management skills. Often they need to cope up with full time jobs in order to take care of their loved ones. In addition to this, they need to also monitor the financial stress that goes hand in hand with care giving. It is true that the life of a caregiver is full of challenges, but there are innumerable rewards as well. In fact, in the care giving process, most caregivers develop a better relationship with the patient they are looking after. Moreover, adequate care giving makes an individual spiritually as well as religiously sound. In a nutshell, care giving leads to stronger relationships and helps in maintaining an optimistic outlook on life. The difficulties that come with care giving may be overcome with effective communication.

The rewards that come with care giving often make up for the hardships associated with it.

Keeping Yourself Safe as a Caregiver

The following areas should always be borne in mind by the caregiver for safety:

1. The five senses

2. Information

3. Sexual behaviors

The sense of hearing: Sound is an important alert for safety. It can indicate that your patient has fallen, that someone is trying to break into the house, things of the sort. The caregiver must always be sound alert. When left alone with your client and the door bell rings, do not open the door if you do not know the person. Some bad person may know that everyone has gone to work and you are left alone with this sick person, and so decides to trick you into opening the door yourself which, of course will not trigger alarms.

The sense of sight: This has earlier on been mentioned under observation skills. Careful observation should be part of the caregiver's skills. Some examples where the sense of sight could be tools for safety include the observation of unusual movement around the house which could be a criminal, observation of your client to see changes in his mood and behavior on time. Take the necessary actions, and save yourself troubles that could arise out of your neglect.

The sense of touch: Always react to any feel of undue wetness. If this is noted on the floor, dry it without waste of time to avoid falls, if it is on the bed, or diaper, change the client to avoid pressure ulcers. Using your sense of touch, always take note of your clients temperature becoming warmer than usual. Could he or she be having a fever?

The sense of smell: This tells you if something is burning which of course should be investigated. Shut off to avoid fire. It may also tell you when your patient is wet.

The sense of taste: This will be mostly used if you are preparing meals for the client.

167

Information: Keep watch for useful information that could affect both your safety and the safety of the caregiver. This could be information on fire around the neighborhood, flood, earthquakes, and the sort. Any information that could hamper your safety or that of your client should be of paramount importance to you.

Sexual Behaviors: Bear it in mind that a lot of caregivers have had issues of sexual assaults in their records and that many of these people are probably innocent. So, in order to keep yourself safe during the care giving job, avoid comments or behaviors that can easily be misunderstood. An example is when changing the diaper of an old man, and you observe his penis, forget your professionalism and start asking him if he was circumcised. Also avoid touches that may be misunderstood as sexual harassment.

<u>More information on keeping yourself safe as a caregiver</u>

Caregivers' minds encircle with questions but with the call of their duty, they forget to distinguish that there are some things which are beyond their limit; they try to achieve them and unfortunately in the process they tend to lose spirit and motivation and thus their mental and physical health deteriorate. Caring for an individual who is suffering from a severe disease can be challenging. In the case of caring for Alzheimer's disease or any related dementia, there is the possibility that the caregiver can become frustrated and irritated. If they are ignored and not treated, they can become depressed and that ultimately can lead to serious consequences for the person the caregivers care for. Thus, it is not only necessary for the person the caregiver is caring for but it is also important for the self-belief and the satisfaction of a caregiver's job.

Why care for a caregiver?

Frustration often arises when a caregiver tries to change some uncontrollable situations and this frustration can even arise from any daily activities like bathing, dressing and eating. When a caregiver is taking care of some serious cases like the bone marrow or cord blood transplant, it can be really stressful. The patient's behavior can also become irritating to caregivers. Examples are when a patient is wandering or repeatedly asking questions, the caregiver has to be patient and overcome their frustration and stress because the fact is that the caregivers are entrusted with the duty of caring for the patient and not the other way round. If you are a caregiver, taking care of yourself is not only about taking out 15 minutes and spending some time with your friends. Rather it is more about finding someone, who will be able to give you an emotional support and can really motivate you to get your fit into the role.

A Caregiver's Life

The caregiver's stress can lead to an emotional and physical strain, thus leading to frustration and anger while taking care of the patient. In some cases, the person may feel guilty thinking that he/she is not able to deliver the best of the care to the patient. There may be feelings of loneliness and exhaustion. These mentioned factors can lead to serious complications, but the good news is that these complications can be avoided.

The warning signs

Some of the signs of frustration are:

- headache
- chest pains
- lack of patience
- stomach cramps
- knot in the throat
- compulsive eating
- shortness of breath
- increased smoking

- desire to strike out

- regular alcohol consumption

For combating all these symptoms it is necessary that a caregiver should respond to an extreme frustration and for doing that, you need the following:

- help yourself to learn the signs and the symptoms
- intervene or calm down physically
- thought modification process can be helpful for reducing your stress
- assertive communication is necessary
- seek help

When you are caring for others, the precautionary steps are different for different diseases. There are even some precautionary steps which you should take for yourself. So make the process easy. It is necessary that you should make some plans that will help both you and the care recipient.

Keeping yourself safe

Caring for yourself should be your first priority because when you are able to love and care for yourself then you can assume the role of a caregiver. Thus watching for the warning signs for the frustration is important as you can intervene with the immediate activity to calm down. Calming down is necessary when there are any tensed situations involving the patient. Trying out these simple processes could be helpful:

- Count one to ten slowly and take few breaths
- Take a brief walk to another room and collect your thoughts
- Any uncontrollable situations should be left for the moment and if possible avoid any self reaction
- You can even try reading, praying, meditating, singing, music or taking a bath
- Practicing relaxing techniques at last for 10 minutes in a day

If possible, try to recall the whole situation and replay in your mind all that happened and what you should have done to make the situation better. This is a very useful too which will help to reduce some of the stress from the job. There are many situations which affect how you feel and there can be feelings of frustration from any such difficult circumstances. If you are able to analyze these situations, and follow the thought patterns which are adaptive in nature then there could be a buildup of self-defense against frustration. Also trying to transform unhealthful thought patterns into adaptive and positive thought patterns can also be useful. Some of the common thought patterns are:

You can take up some negative thoughts and multiply it with something else, for example when you are becoming ready to take the patient to the doctor, the car breaks down and you tend to think that something always goes wrong whenever you are taking him/her outside.

You tend to overlook good situations and hardly ever think about motivation like "I can do more", rather you capitalize on the bad moments.

Sometimes you may even jump to a conclusion without being aware of the facts. You tend to think of others thinking negatively of you and your duties and thus you unconsciously show that in your actions.

As said earlier, take pride in your job, motivate yourself and make the most of the moment. Carry out your duties in such a way that the client will see you as the "ideal caregiver".

One of the most important things for the caregiver is to have the right amount of sleep because deprivation of sleep can cause moodiness and thus it might affect the care giving process for the patient. Quality sleep is important and it is not just about the hours you sleep, it is more about the requirement of the body. Since care giving job may involve getting up early in the morning and remaining alert throughout the day, perhaps you need more sleep. In many cases, the caregiving duties are split into shifts like night and day shift. When you are not on 'duty', make sure to take enough rest. If it happens that you are the only one that does all the shifts, ask for help, so as to rest yourself and be healthy to meet the demands of the job.

Some of the common ways of decreasing your stress as a caregiver could be explained in a nutshell, like the following:

1. Arrange a meeting with your family when a loved one is diagnosed. This will enable each family member to decide on how much they can contribute towards a paid caregiver. That way, you will not suffer because you are the only one at home with the senior.

2. Self-care is necessary because if the caregiver becomes ill, the entire care giving process is disrupted. If the caregiver is not well, then it is better to handover the task to someone else who's trustworthy, someone from the family or from outside.

3. It is necessary to take care of the stress levels which you are facing in the process of caring for the patient. There could be some early warning signs for potential problem and it is important to check them out so as to maintain the care giving process.

4. Meeting physical needs: When you are taking care of someone, it is important for you to be 100% fit and sound and this can be possible when you are consuming proper healthy food, having sufficient rest and have time for recreation and relaxation.

5. Honesty counts: If you feel that you are not being able to meet the mental and physical demands of the care of the patient, being honest with your inabilities will certainly help you.

6. Making legal and financial plans on the forefront. It is necessary to take care of the advance directories like Health Care Surrogate, Living Will and Power

of Attorney will help you to take care of the business in advance.

7. Realistic approach: Be hopeful but keep yourself grounded with the realities of the moment. It will help you to reduce your stress up to certain level when you are able to balance the hopefulness and realities relayed to the condition of the patient.

8. 100% Not possible: it is wise to accept the fact, that there can be certain situations where you may not be able to provide 100% perfect care to your loved one or whoever is the patient. Be cautious and never overdo anything because that might cause problems to the patient and thereby enhancing your stress level.

9. Avoid guilty feeling unnecessarily: Learning to say NO is not a guilt and there could even be times when you won't hear the word THANK YOU, however, be patient and learn to deal with feelings of grief and anger.

10. Praise yourself: you are not a super hero or a saint, but as a human being you have given your best and you have been able to handle numerous responsibilities with great deal of stress. So, praise yourself even if no one else does.

Communication skills

Good communication with the patient or to someone related with the patient is very important. It helps you to know what is expected of you and makes you feel safe to express yourself so that others could understand your limits and needs. The process of Assertive Communication is different from Passive Communication or Aggressive communication.

"Passive communication is a form of expression that is ineffective and maladaptive. Those with a passive communication style are generally afraid of confrontation and do not feel they have the right to make their wishes and desires known. This style of communication can lead to feelings of anxiety, anger, depression and helplessness and is common among those with social anxiety disorder (SAD)."[3] "Passive communication is based on compliance and hopes to avoid confrontation at all costs. In this mode we don't talk much, question even less, and actually do very little. We just don't want to rock the boat. Passives have learned that it is safer not to react and better to disappear than

---

[3] http://socialanxietydisorder.about.com/od/glossaryp/g/passive.htm

to stand up and be noticed."[4] From the descriptions given about passive communication, it is clear that this is not the type of communication that the care giver needs.

"Aggressive communication always involves manipulation. We may attempt to make people do what we want by inducing guilt (hurt) or by using intimidation and control tactics (anger). Covert or overt, we simply want our needs met - and right now! Although there are a few arenas where aggressive behavior is called for (i.e., sports or war), it will never work in a relationship. Ironically, the more aggressive sports rely heavily on team members and rational coaching strategies. Even war might be avoided if we could learn to be more assertive and negotiate to solve our problems"[5]

Having seen the above two types of communication, we may want to look at assertive communication. "The most effective and healthiest form of communication is the assertive style. It's how we naturally express ourselves when our self-esteem is intact, giving us the confidence to

---

[4] http://www.angelfire.com/az2/webenglish/commstyles.html

[5] http://www.angelfire.com/az2/webenglish/commstyles.html

communicate without games and manipulation. When we are being assertive, we work hard to create mutually satisfying solutions. We communicate our needs clearly and forthrightly. We care about the relationship and strive for a win/win situation. We know our limits and refuse to be pushed beyond them just because someone else wants or needs something from us. Surprisingly, assertive is the style most people use least."[6]

Some of the important keys to assertive communications are:

- Respect your own feelings, desires and needs
- Speak about your feelings without any hesitation, shame or humiliation
- Use 'I' statements rather than 'You' statements
- Use words like "Its important to…" rather than using "should" in your statements

When you feel that that it will not be possible for you to continue as a caregiver, then it is better to accept this fact because that will not be favorable to you alone but to the

---

[6] ibid

patient as well. It is wise to discuss your needs along with the family members and friends and you will be able to share the care giving responsibility. It is quite natural that people will not realize when you need help or assistance. Therefore you should take the initiative to ask for help and express your needs. If someone offers you help don't refuse because there could be errands or task when you need to attend to.

<u>More information on communication</u>

When your loved one is suffering from diseases like Alzheimer or Dementia, it can be really a difficult task to get the right communication. It is usually very difficult to convey the message across their senses and if they are not able to perceive, that you cannot blame them because the decreased level of perception is consistent with these types of patients. There can however, be certain times of the days which can be worse or better; when they will be able to understand what you want to communicate and respond accordingly. There can also be times when they sit still and it will be like talking to a stone idol. Whatever may be the case it is necessary to understand their needs and demand, understand them and communicate effectively. So here are 5 positive communication techniques which will help to get your message right across towards the patient and thereby fulfill the caregiver's duty towards the patient.

- The first and foremost thing that is necessary is to put ourselves in their shoes. That is essential because unless you are able to understand their problems and inabilities, you won't be able to take off the righteous methods to communicate with them. The person suffering from dementia needs to be knowledgeable about his/her disease and that should not be done by force. There is no need to give them any "gentle reminder" or "correction" because that could be psychologically damaging. It is better to congratulate them rather than correcting them as it will be easier to cope up with the situation. So improve this part of communication with them and offer them with the support and validation they want.

- Another important factor which you need to keep in mind is to place the right kind of communication with the health care providers. It is necessary to convey all the problems and difficulties the patient faces. Recognize and demonstrate wellness habits of the patient to the doctor. You need to recognize all the signs and symptoms of the common chronic illness and have to abide with the process of treatment and the lifestyle changes that is required for the managing the chronic illness.

- Using effective communication techniques and strategies for the older adults and recognizing and responding to the challenging behaviors of the older patients. If you are not well aware of the communication techniques, you can plan a doctor's visit and learn communication practical skills from them to conduct an effective communication with the doctors, nurses, home health workers and health care providers.

- Allow the elder person to express their feelings because it will help them to disclose some hidden feelings of significant loss. If they don't express they will tend to develop sadness and grief and may in turn lead to more deterioration of their health. Sit with them and try to make a space so that they don't hesitate to share their inner feelings.

- Since an elder patient has various life experiences, it is important for them to allow the person with thoughts and it is necessary to listen and respect them.

Try out these techniques as they may be challenging at times but it's worth the effort.

Cultural Sensitivity in Home Care giving

Performing a routine task for the toddlers or patients is similar to what we generally do for our own family. The point is to be at the demarcation line where care giver services are to be peddled but keeping the professionalism intact. Caregivers need to be aware of cultural differences that why I have chosen to address it in this book. Conflicts should be avoided because of cultural differences, that is why the caregiver should do an "assessment" of the client at the beginning of her job to know what the client likes and what she/he does not; to know what he believes in or does not. This will encourage a smoother communication and help build a therapeutic relationship faster. Listening carefully and respectfully to the values and beliefs of the patients and respecting them in your day to day activity is what is referred to as cultural sensitivity.

Culture is referred to as "the way of life of the people". I knew this definition from my high school so I do not know the source. So, when we are saying that the caregiver should be culturally sensitive, we are saying that the caregiver should respect the way of life of her client! Culture is made of values, beliefs and practices and they are shared by some group, children inherit culture from their elder ones and it lasts throughout adulthood.

Advantages of cultural sensitivity

- Person becomes competent and confident
- A stronger connection with the client and the family members.
- Families share a trusting relationship with the caregiver.
- Effective meeting with families and children
- Expansion of knowledge
- Avoidance of conflicts

Follow these simple tips and avoid conflicts with the patient:

- Reflect on the care giving practices and analyze the things which are being done or performed
- Observe the interactions of the close ones and relatives with the patient
- Differences may arise with the relatives but it is better to acknowledge them as it will reduce anxiety and confusion.
- Ask for more information and learn about the relatives and close one's perspective and clarify every point of view. This will help to handle situations or any issue arising from the patient's abnormal behaviors arising out of cultural sensitivity.

Communication is the best way to negotiate with any differences arising out of cultural sensitivity. So check out these few tips:

- Build a trusting relationship with the close ones and relatives of the patient
- Determine the level of commitment necessary to resolve the problem
- Identify problems in words and decide the plan of action

Escorting and Transporting Your Patient

Dealing with patients requires a lot of care and professional expertise. Escorting and transporting a patient implies monitoring the mental and physical state of the person during the whole journey. A person who is escorting and transporting a patient is fully responsible for observing any signs of discomfort or anxiety during the journey. In the event of any kind of discomfort or anxiety the care giver should take all the required steps to alleviate the cause of discomfort with the help of their skills and expertise.

Escorting a patient should not be confused with accompanying a patient to a destination. Both tasks are different from one another and they should not be confused. A person's relative or friend may accompany a person whereas escorting a patient is a professional role and hence this task is generally conducted by professional care givers like health or social care professionals.

Before transporting a patient the personnel who is handling the patient should make sure that the client is properly dressed for the occasion. If the destination is the doctor's office or the mall, it is important to dress the senior with a cardigan to guard against the coldness usually associated with these areas because of the air conditioner. While in the car, make sure all buckles and button have been pressed. If the person is on a wheel chair, makes sure the knots holding the wheelchair to the floor of the transport has been knotted. If it is a car, make sure the seat belt has been put on. Whatever the case, your security, as well as the security of the client are of paramount importance.

Before escorting the patient the care giver should be familiar with the appropriate destination well in advance. The anticipated time of return should also be discussed with the patient and in the case of delays the mobile and phone numbers of the concerned people or units should be with him or her.

Escorting and transporting a person are generally for the purposes of attending an appointment e.g. to a doctor's chamber, court or housing department, requiring an assessment outside the hospital for e.g. home, transferring from one place to another or taking the patient to an inpatient department of a medical unit.

A person who is escorting and transporting a patient should be aware of the medical history and the clinical condition of the patient. There should be provision for water as while traveling the patient's mouth may become dry. Toilet and food breaks should be ensured in consultation with the patient throughout the journey. Medication should be provided as prescribed and if the medication should be taken with food there should be a stop for food during the journey.

After the escort and on return the care giver must make an entry in the patient's record. The record should contain elaborate details identifying the reason for the escort, the patient's behavior and the outcome of the escort. The details of any accidents or incidents that occurred during the escort should also be recorded in the patient's records. In home care giving, if there were no incidences, there will be no need to make any records.

The above mentioned points should be taken into consideration when escorting and transporting a patient. They require a lot of care and attention and more importantly the understanding and love of the care giver who is taking care of them.

Fire and Safety Preparedness

Every year there are innumerable residential fires that lead to damage of property or loss of life. Well damage to property can be recovered but what if someone loses his or life. As an ideal caregiver your prime responsibility lies in adapting fire and safety measures and protecting the client in case a fire breaks out. By adhering to a fire and safety measures and being vigilant a homecare giver can lower the risk of a fire break out to a considerable extent.

Some of the probable reasons of a fire break out are smoking, cooking, and a couple of other fire hazards. Let us now take a closer look at how an ideal home care giver can prevent fire break outs from taking place.

Cooking

- While answering a phone call or stepping out of the house the burner should be turned off
- While handling hot pans and pots oven mitts should be used

- While preparing a meal, the cooking oil should be heated in low flame
- Avoid putting flammable towels as well as mitts on the stove

Smoking

- The lighter and old matches should be disposed
- The matches, cigars as well as cigarettes should be kept at a safe place
- Make sure the patient never lies down while smoking or consuming alcohol
- Dropped butts needs to be disposed in large tin cans at the earliest
- For the elimination of ashes, large ashtrays should be used

Additional precautions:

- Ask a professional to clean the fireplace chimney frequently
- Opt for extension cords that come with circuit breakers. Avoid overloading the circuit breaker
- The electrical cords should not hang from the book shelves
- The electrical panel should be inspected on a routine basis. You can appoint an expert electrician for this purpose.
- A good quality security system needs to be set up in your house
- The yard as well as the house should be well lighted
- If you are escorting the patient to the hospital, make sure there is someone to keep an eye on the house

- The yard, garage as well as home needs to be free of rubbish as well as combustible items
- There needs to be a provision for a fire extinguisher in the house
- The windows as well as the doors needs to be free from obstructions for easy and safe exit
- A smoke detector needs to be installed in the house
- The electric smoke alarms should be checked on a consistent basis
- Try cleaning the alarms after every six months
- The battery of the alarms needs to be charged at least once in a year
- Close the doors and windows closed while the patient is asleep as this provides some prevention against fire

It is hoped that the aforementioned suggestions will help an ideal home care giver in preventing his/her patient as well as other members of the family from the disasters caused due to a fire break out.

Phone Etiquette for a Home Caregiver

Telephone is a part of daily activity and for a caregiver, it is part of the requirements of the job. Since it is a part of the areas where caregivers have to walk and talk, there are certain things which are essential to follow as a part of the telephone etiquette. In every good care giving course, telephone etiquette is a part of the curriculum. This is because it is certainly important to prevent treating the elderly or the people on the other line rudely or abruptly when communicating. The caregiver helps in conveying any emergency problems to the doctor or to the family members. In the process, there could be the possibility of the caregiver showing bad manners while speaking on the telephone to address the patient's problem. That is why good etiquette is needed.

There could also be the tendency to be too short or become 'the salesperson' in most of the telephone calls. Have you ever had an experience with someone who is just rude on the phone? Or someone that wants you to explain things hundred times up to the amount of frustration? If you have had any of these experiences, then you will understand why the caregiver needs to adopt good phone manners. Politeness and simplicity is not the only manners needed in conducting proper phone etiquette, there are certain other things as well.

Talking of the proper way to answer the telephone, except "hello" nothing is accepted as the proper way to start addressing the other person on the phone when answering from a non-business phone. Using words like "Yes" is considered inappropriate in telephone etiquette. The individual calling tends to draw a quick conclusion and therefore the person sounds cold and aloof and will hesitate to communicate effectively. As a caregiver, when you are calling someone, it is better to address them properly and generally it is better to start this way: "May I speak to Mr._____ please," and in case the person who is being asked for is not present in the house then a proper way to tell "I am sorry Mr._____ is not available at this time, Can I take a message?" Don't utter anything abrupt like "NO" because that reflects your negativity on the caller.

Even if someone calls the number of your client mistakenly, it is better not to hang up, but to politely say "I am sorry, but this is a wrong number."

When you are making a telephone call to the doctor or to the relatives of the patient at odd times like late in the night (Any call after 8:30 pm is considered late), it is necessary to be patient and courteous while describing the person's emergency. In case of wrong dialing of the number, expressing apology is a must. When you are not with the patient, and you are communicating him/her on the telephone, it is important to be patient and calm with your voice to get across the message to your patient.

In a nutshell, here are few of the Phone etiquette tips as a home caregiver.

- Be very calm, calculated and patient on the phone
- Remember that you are representing your client, so be very professional
- Do not pass out your bad emotions to persons on the other line
- Dialing wrong numbers demand prompt apology and not hanging up abruptly
- Calling any business nearing the closing time should be avoided if possible
- When you are calling any health professionals or doctor, keep your calls short and informative as they are generally busy people

PART TWO: Common cases found in home care giving and how to deal with them.

<u>Ten ways to prevent falls for seniors in the home</u>

Do you know that nearly fifty percent of the falls experienced by seniors take place in the home itself? Well, there isn't any need to get worried as I have some good news for you: all you need to do is bring about a couple of improvements and modifications in the senior's home. Also following the suggestions included here will help to prevent your seniors for innumerable common hazards that may lead to disabling or in rare cases fatal falls. These suggestions are sure to help seniors lead a safe life.

With aging, the risk for falling increases because their senses dim and nervous systems tends to deteriorate. Elderly people often suffer from weakened vision and the balance mechanism in their ears becomes less accurate. The sedentary lifestyle of theirs may lead to muscle loss, thereby leading to falls. In seniors, even a minor fall may at times lead to fractured bones.

How to make our home a safe to live in place for seniors:

- Bathroom…a risk prone place! That's true…falls are more commonly to take place in bathrooms…hence it would be advisable on your part to set up bath benches in your bathroom so that seniors are at a lower risk to slip. Also arrange for toilet risers, toilet safety frames, grab bars and tub and shower treads. Well, I guess you get me...I intend to say that you need to make your bathroom slip resistant. How? Well, that's a good question, I must say! To begin with, for adding steady support in case of slippery situations, you need to install non-slip strips on the shower floor or tub. In addition to this, you need to place non-skid mats on the floors of your bathroom. You can also look for garb bars that have been approved by the ADA.

- Falls among seniors can also be a result of dim light or poor vision, particularly in areas such as basements and stairways. So how can you avoid that? Well, your first step lies in installing brighter light bulbs throughout your house. It would be better, if you opt for bulbs with greater longevity as they'll never burn out at a time you need them the most. Opt for bright lights for your bedrooms, bathrooms, stairwells and hallways. While new fluorescent bulbs have a greater longevity as compared to the conventional incandescents, yet despite this fact some may not like the light that they deliver.

- Go for motion-sensor switches which turn on lights automatically while entering an area. You can also go for light switches which glow; hence you can look for them easily during the dark.

- Make sure you install nightlights close to the floor for lowering the chances of falling or tripping while you need to pay a visit to the bathroom during the nighttime.

- Another way through which you can help seniors from tripping is by clearing off the debris from hallways, stairs and walkways.

- Try removing the scatter rugs. If you fail to do so, then it would be ideal on your part to secure the rags to the floor using heavy duty and double-sided tape. You don't have to wander hither and thither in search of these, simply walk up to any hardware store and order for one!

- You can play safe with the stairways if you paint a white strip (ensure the measurement is somewhere around two inch) on the top of the each step's edge. Try using a gritty paint as it helps your seniors in staying more surefooted while they move up as well as down. This isn't all...seniors are at a greater risk to fall from the carpeted steps as well. But you can avoid this problem if you use white colored non-skid tape.

- Keep an eye on the electrical cords and make sure they don't obstruct any foot paths. Don't overcrowd the cabinets, bookcases and shelves. And make sure they aren't too high. This approach will prevent the seniors from using a stepladder or stool while taking off things from the cabinets, bookcases and shelves. Try placing a chair or bench close to the entrances as this will provide you a secure and handy place for setting down bags, or sitting down while slipping your shoes on as well as off.

- Get their vision and hearing checked on a routine basis. In other words, start the checkups even before noticing problems. Consult with the doctor about the drug therapy for ensuring that after taking it you won't feel dizzy.

- Elderly people should avoid standing up quickly as this may make you feel dizzy and probably fall. Prior to standing, try wiggling your feet and toes and swing your legs, if needed. Try exercising on a routine basis as this helps in strengthening your muscles as well as improving your agility. However, prior to this make sure you consult your doctor.

- Before standing up, try moving enough so that your blood pressure and heart rate increases. And last but not the least elderly people should limit their consumption of alcohol.

With aging, the risk for falling goes on increasing. It is true that most of the falls lead to minor injuries, but at the same time nearly ten to fifty percent lead to fractures as well as other serious injuries. Falls may take place anywhere, but a senior may more commonly experience it in the home. To be more specific, falls are likely to take place while getting out or climbing the bathtub.

In addition to elderly people, people suffering from weakness in legs or feet, problems with balance and walking, arthritis, particularly in the knee, problems with vision or hearing, dementia, low blood pressure, dehydration also run at a greater risk of developing falls. In a nutshell, the more risk factor a person is prone to, the more are their chances of falls.

Prevention of falls for Seniors (contd)

Falls are one of the common occurrences in a person's life as they grow older. There are many reasons that can cause a fall for seniors. It is indeed a big problem and falls can sometime prove to be life threatening. There are many people who are affected badly by the falls resulting into permanent injuries. Injuries that can result out of falls are broken bones, head injuries and even accidents that harm the interior body parts. Head injuries can be more damaging than any other falls and can cause problems like memory loss or blood clot.

Falls for the seniors can be easily prevented if we use some of the prevention tips that help to cut down the accidents. Let's look at some of these valuable tips:

a) Enroll the seniors for an exercise program: Now, body fitness is a big thing when it comes to preventing falls. Seniors can enroll for fitness programs that would make them physically fit thus reducing the chances of a fall. One can on the yoga or Tai Chi classes as they are neither very taxing on the body nor provide very tough regimens to follow. Fat and unfit bodies are more prone to falls and the only way to avoid these is regular exercise. Exercise can also help to reduce fat and provide the necessary fitness to legs and hands. It is better to practice the yoga moves or exercises that help to improve the strength of the leg muscles. You can seek the help of an expert or doctor in order to guide you choose the right exercise program.

b) Safe home to live at: Falls at home is a common thing and most of the falls occur at or homes. You must remove the objects that can cause you or the seniors at home to trip. Things like books, shoes and other objects can cause real problems for the seniors as there is a fear of tripping over them. Use tapes to stop the rugs from slipping over. Try to put the daily use items in the closet and keep them at a height that you or the seniors can reach easily. Install the grab bars beside the toilet or bath tub. The mats that one uses should not be slippery and try to wear the shoes that are not slippery and provide a good holding on the ground.

c) Get an eye check: You need to ensure that the seniors have a proper vision and the only way to so is to get it checked by the doctor. The doctor can provide glasses or lenses that would improve the vision if there are any such problems. It often happens that seniors keep on wearing the same glasses for long without getting their eyes checked. Now this is a sure way of getting falls. Proper and regular eye checkup is necessary for the aging eyes.

d) Get your medicines checked: You need to get the medicines of seniors checked by the doctor as they may be taking medicines that make them drowsy. You need to be a little more careful about the medicines to avoid the falls for seniors.

The care of a person in the early stages of Alzheimer's disease

Alzheimer's is a common form of dementia in which a person faces problem with their memory or thought process. Memory or thought related problems can affect anyone irrespective of their age or sex and when this starts hampering daily life activities then this can mean real trouble. The changes can even affect the personality or the mood of the patient. The number of dementia related cases is somewhere near 4 million and out of this $2/3^{rd}$ suffers from the problem of Alzheimer's disease.

It is often seen that we forget about an incident that might have occurred only a few moments back but this is not the soul symptom of being affected with something as serious as Alzheimer's. The former case may be a simple problem of a temporary memory failure where the brain fails to recollect information. The symptoms of Alzheimer's are divided into two broad categories: Early stage and late stage. In the early stage, the patient faces the frequent loss in memory (mostly the ones that are related to the recent events and conversations). We even get to see problems like repeating questions, problem with speaking a language, writing and even using a few objects. Depression and changes in the personality can also occur and there are also problems with spatial orientation while walking or driving. These problems keep on increasing with time and take an acute shape and this is what forms the symptoms for the later stage where people face almost complete memory loss. For instance, they forget why they have come to a particular place or why they are walking etc.

There are no straight treatments available for the problem of Alzheimer's and only proper care can make the lives of the patient's easier. It is really a challenging task to take care of a patient with Alzheimer's disease and this can at times prove to be tougher than one can think. A caregiver would face new problems every day and they have to adapt themselves to the fast changing demands of the patient. The behavior pattern of the patient changes and the caregiver needs to make a lot of changes in their caretaking procedure to get acquainted to the new set of demands. Here, we are going to look at the things that can make your job of taking care of a person in the early stages of Alzheimer's a little easy.

After your family member or loved one is diagnosed Alzheimer's, you need to start making changes in your lifestyle and the place you reside, so as to make things easier for the person. Changes are necessary in order to create an environment where the patient would be physically safe and at the same time would feel comfortable. You need to restructure the social lives of the person as it won't remain normal with every passing day. The environment of the home needs to change so as one needs to understand that things won't remain the same anymore. The ways of communication also needs to change and development of new ways of communication should be emphasized upon. For instance, one needs to have prior scheduling for visits to the patient in order to avoid surprise, but this doesn't mean that one needs to snap all social contacts with the Alzheimer's patient. One also needs to make a proper structure of the daily activities that are to be performed by the daily living. One also needs to help out the patient make social contact on a regular basis. You need to set up a safe environment in the home so that the patient does not meet with any accidents at home.

The condition of the patient deteriorates as the days pass and one should understand that the patient becomes emotionally fragile. The emotional support needs to come from the side of the caregiver and this can create a sense of well being in the patient. Even emotional support help to allay the fears and anxiety that build up in the mind of the people who suffer from Alzheimer's. It is better not to use logic in order to alleviate the fear in these patients as they lose their capacity of rational thinking. The risks of accidents and injuries would increase with time, so it is better to be always prepared for them. It is better to rearrange the house to avoid any types of untowardly incidences.

You need to be sensitive towards the patient as there are going to problems that can make your job tougher. If you want to inform the patient about the diagnosis then it is better to do that in a roundabout manner. Do not directly tell the patient that they suffer from the problem of Alzheimer's and instead tell them that it has something to do with their memory problem or anything better that comes to your mind. You should be patient enough while dealing with the queries of the patient and if you are performing a task that the patient is supposed to perform then try to explain to them why you are doing it.

You need to have a positive attitude towards seeing improvement in the patient and should not get bogged down by the initial setbacks. Patients who are in the early stage of Alzheimer's would get worse as they move to the late stages, so one should be ready to expect worse things. If you are taking care of an Alzheimer's patient then you need to communicate with the patient in a way that they can rely and have faith on you. Be supportive to the patient not only when they show up the negative traits but also appreciate if he does anything new or good. You need to understand that these patients are going to have behavioral problem but you also need to be ready to cope up with the same.

Taking care of the Alzheimer's patients is certainly not an easy task and one needs to take good care of oneself in order to provide the best support to the patients.

The Care Of a Person in the Late Stages of Alzheimer's Disease

Alzheimer's and its late stages require a complete different approach in the care of the patient. The care does not get restricted to providing emotional support and taking care of the simple needs but it now shifts to a more complex environment. You need to take round the clock care of the patient and there is hardly any room for leaving the patient alone. In the later stages of the disease, it progresses in a disorderly fashion and this is why there is a need to take care of the patient in a proper way. This time is very crucial for the caregivers or the people who take carte of their Alzheimer inflicted loved ones. It is very challenging to take care of the patients who are in the late stages of Alzheimer's disease. It is often seen that a caregiver gets so attached with performing their daily duties but this is the time when they need to accept the bitter reality that death is a reality that is not very far away from their loved ones. The sense of bereavement can at times make the caregiver mentally weak but they have to gather themselves in order to perform their duties properly till the last breath of their loved one.

One should understand that despite the best care and treatment their loved ones are slowly nearing death. The late stage of Alzheimer attacks the patient so badly that they are not even in a position to communicate properly and they are completely dependent on the caregiver. They are bedridden and look forward to their caregivers even for their daily requirements. This is the time when they lose all their memory and do not remember even their loved ones with whom they might have spent happy days even a few years back. They become more and more dependent on their caregivers as they are not even in a position to verbally let their needs or requirements known.

You must know the fact that at the late stage the patient of Alzheimer's is not at all in a position to sit, talk, walk or eat and they even cannot make any sense of the world around them. This is the time when the caregivers go through a testing time. They have to take care of daily activities of the patient like bathing, feeding, toileting and dressing. You have to be in a position to take complete care of the patients and this is the time when the caregivers also need to be mentally as well as physically fit.

Memory loss in the Alzheimer's disease doesn't mean that the patient loses their feelings. They experience normal feelings like fear, sadness, peace, lonely, loved etc. Now, you are the only person who can provide solace to the patient and you are also the one who can allay all their fears and discomfort. It is best to not leave the patient alone while they are awake as they would not be able to communicate their feelings but their bodily gestures may provide you with some hints.

In the late stage one can even look at the other options for patient care as it is not always possible to keep the patient at home. Looking at the physical safety needs of the patient or the need for an advanced treatment, one has to find a hospital or care centre where the patient can be under 24 hour monitoring. The decision to keep a last stage patient at home means that the caregiver has to have a lot of mental strength and complete family support without which there is no way a person can stand the jitters. If you are keeping your loved one at home then you need to make a world of changes in the way you have been living and also the place where your loved one lives. The patient's needs for the changes are to be first jotted down so that you do everything to make the adjustment of the patient pretty easy. It has been often seen that the people who are in the early stage do not face problems with adjustments, but patients in the late stage can feel completely lost with minor changes. Well this is attributed to the fact that the late stage patients do not have the ability to remember even the smallest changes around them.

Here are a few things that would help you to understand whether you are in any position to take care of an Alzheimer's patient:

a) See if you are in a position to take a 24 hour care of the patient or not. This is very important as you need to understand that Alzheimer's patients in their last stages require complete support even for their smallest daily activities.

b) Find out whether your room has the provision for a hospital bed, Commode or wheel chair. This is because the patient needs to move as less as possible.

c) Is there a proper transportation support so that the patient can be moved whenever any emergency crops up?

d) You also need to judge whether you possess the necessary stamina to lift or carry your loved one or not.

The last stage of Alzheimer's completely cripples a person both mentally as well as physically, so you have to mentally prepare yourself to be close to a person who cannot even communicate his daily needs in a proper way. There is a bid difference in reading about the difficulties and actually experiencing the same from close quarters. The care giver has to be very attentive to catch even the smallest gestures of the patient to understand their requirements. One has to be so habituated with the patient that there is not even a single movement of the patient that misses one's eyes. One needs to learn some soothing techniques like massage, fragrance, music and touch so as to provide a holistic comfort system to the system. The people who perform the job of a caretaker should themselves have a support system as they are the ones who have to witness the agonizing days of the patient before they finally expire. If you are a caregiver then you must learn to get proper grip over your emotions and become mentally strong.

Autism And How To Care For An Autistic Patient

We have very often come across the term "Autism" in our daily lives. There are many of us who have heard the term however we are still not sure about what it actually implies. In general autism is a persuasive developmental disorder that impairs a child's normal development of language, communication and social interaction skills. Many are still unaware of the actual causes of the disorder and its treatment options. The subject of autism has been one of constant research and there have been many scientific breakthroughs in its diagnosis and treatment process.

Autism is a brain disorder that deals with an abnormal self absorption with oneself. It is marked with communication disorders and a short attention span. Autism involves restricted and repetitive behavior in patients and the signs of autism begin when a child is three years. There are two other autism related disorders which in medical terms are called Asperger Syndrome and Pervasive Developmental Disorder - Not Otherwise Specified (PDD-NOS). Both of these disorders fall under the category of Autism Spectrum Disorders or ASD.

- Asperger Syndrome: The patient displays significant difficulties in social interaction coupled with a series of restricted and repetitive behavioral patterns. Those afflicted with autism are physically clumsy and they frequently use a typical form of language.

- Pervasive Developmental Disorder - Not Otherwise Specified (PDD-NOS): PDD-NOS is a milder autism disorder. In this disorder the patient does not suffer from all the symptoms of autism.

Autism and both the Autism Spectrum Diseases are complicated neurodevelopment disorders and its causes are still not definitely proven. A lot of research is still on and medically doctors are of the opinion that autism is a genetic disorder. There are some rare cases where autism is caused by some birth defect causing agents. There are some that are of the opinion that certain after effects of vaccines may be the cause of autism however such hypotheses have no scientific evidence and have not been convincingly proven.

One can easily identify the early symptoms of autism in children. Autistic children display comprehension and language development impairments. They respond poorly to name and they have deficient non verbal communication for example they lack appropriate emotional gestures, ignore people, prefer to be alone, lack of pointing and problems with following a point, lack of social interaction skills with others etc. The indicators of autistic behavior in very young children are no babble, pointing or gestures by the 12th month, no single word by the 18th month, no two word spontaneous phrase by the 24th month and any loss of language or social skill at any age. Autistic children either ignore or have a very friendly attitude with adults. They tend to prefer loneliness and they love being in their own imaginary world. They prefer solitary activities and they have a social imagination that they generally do not share with others. They have social impairments and they are over sensitive to moods and touch. They tend to play repetitive games with toys, for example lining up of objects and the turning on and off of light switches despite repeated scolding.

Autism can also be present in adults and normally the Asperger Syndrome disorder sometimes transits into adulthood too. This type of autism is called classic autism and there are many people who are unaware of these traits in adults. Autistic adults function independently and on most occasions also obtain college degrees. Psychiatrists and pediatricians in the past and sometimes even today are reluctant to pronounce adults as autistic out of compassion for their parents. These adults have poor living skills and are either reclusive or eccentric. They have a level of social awkwardness and they tend to prefer being on their own. They may be unable to care for themselves and fail to comprehend the social behavior of others. They are generally obsessed with a particular subject and they tend to bring the topic of any discussion back to their interests. They tend to become angry if they cannot do what they want or if they are stuck in a schedule that disinterests them. They are generally not empathetic and do not understand the emotions of others except their own. People with autism also have problems with keeping the track of time when they are engaged in activities that they like doing the most. They tend to stack and organize things on shelves and they love to do solitary activities. Autistic adults have a lack of emotional control and though their emotional outbursts may not be like a child it can be very irritating to any normal person or bystander.

One cannot physically identify a person with autistic traits however when communicating with a patient one may be able to ascertain the levels of autism as its levels differ from individual to individual. Some physical characteristic of autism may include:

- The face has low muscle tone
- The eyes may be large with pupil dilation
- The skin is pale
- The tendency of banging one's head
- The tendency of slapping one's ears
- The motor skills of the patient are impaired.

Children with autistic tendencies have problems painting, coloring, solving jigsaw puzzles and doing other normal classroom activities like normal children. They are very slow in development than other normal children. These characteristics may differ from one child to another and in most cases therapy can make a difference to treatment in these patients. The following are some important real facts about autism that are beneficial to understand the disorder more clearly:

- Autism occurs in one of every 150 births
- After cerebral palsy and mental retardation it is the third most common developmental disability in the world.

- It occurs more often than the diseases of childhood cancer, cystic fibrosis, and multiple sclerosis.
- The disorder begins before the age of three years.
- Experimental regimens of diet coupled with mineral and vitamin supplements are successful as therapy and treatments are done through medical interventions and behavioral therapy.
- In many cases insurance companies do not cover or recognize various treatments for autism
- Significant improvements have been observed with the recent treatment and medical therapies.
- Both autistic children and adults live a normal life span

Autism is a spectrum disorder and the care of autistic patients differ from individual to individuals. There are no laboratory tests to confirm autism and one can identify its symptoms through a detailed developmental case history of the child and clinical examination. A psychological evaluation should be carried out by a professional to confirm whether a person is autistic or not. The psychologist generally conducts a series of autism screening tests to determine whether a patient is autistic or not. There is no hard and fast rule that autistic patients need to be treated with medicines. There are many effective strategies that can help one with dealing with these patients.

One should keep a notebook or a detailed journal about the patient. One should always track the developmental history of the patient. One may be asked to keep a set of questionnaires which will ask about the behavior and development of the patient.

Writing the daily developments of the patient will help one successfully keep track of the patient. Moreover one can also observe what can work and what cannot work with the patient. This notebook and journal comes in handy when the patient may be difficult to handle at times. It helps to identify the patterns for difficult times and the triggers for the problems that may be faced by the patient.

One should have a positive attitude when dealing with an autistic patient. There may be some days when the patient responds positively to therapy and on some days there may be reverse reactions. One should not be de motivated and discouraged with the results. One should be patient and have a very understanding attitude towards the autistic child or person. In the process one can also find out what thinks work for the patient and what does not. It helps in the long run as the person becomes aware of what he needs to avoid.

The autistic patient may have fixations like making repeated noises, staring at turning wheels etc. There may be some obsessions with objects, TV programs, animals etc. Control and tolerance of this behavior within controlled parameters can be a powerful tool that can help in the patient's educational, emotional and social instruction. One can relate to the interests of the patient and thus gain the confidence of the patient. This leads to acceptance of new things especially in children who suffer from autistic disorders. Using this time with the patient can help one relate and hence connect with the patient on a higher level.

When caring for an autistic child or patient one can find support in the company of other autistic caretakers and hence get essential help. There are many trusted individuals who can provide childcare and advice on how to deal with patients having the same disorder.

One can check with one State Health Department to check there are special health departments that can take care of patients with similar health care needs. One can also resort to visual stimuli. Most autistic children are visually oriented and very often they love to communicate with the use of sign language and pointing out to pictures in a special book that may be put together to help them communicate. Even an autistic child who speaks may be able to communicate better with the help of visual stimulus. If one wants to teach the child something the use of a picture book comes in handy and the child responds well to the technique. Some autistic children can repeat verbal instructions word to word however they are not able to convert their thoughts into actions. Pictures very often can help them to that and hence it is a successful mechanism for teaching autistic children. Autistic individuals often have poor auditory processing skills. As a result of this they often do not understand what people are saying to them. They tend to hear the words but they do not understand what the words actually mean. Very often the person's lack of understanding can lead to confusion and utter frustration to others. Very often this may also escalate into behavioral problems. Picture visual aids can also help them to a considerable extent.

Sometimes an autistic child may demonstrate behavior problems at school but not at home, or vice versa. For example, the parent may have already developed a strategy to tackle and stop such behavior at home, but the teacher is unaware of this strategy and the child continues to be troublesome. In such cases the parent and the teacher should interact on a regular basis to solve this problem in the child. If the child's behavior is bad at school but not at home there are many possible reasons for this behavior such as a lack of consistency. There are can be physical causes and it has been observed that cleaning solvents and florescent classroom lighting can trigger negative responses in autistic children. The janitors very often use powerful chemicals to clean classrooms and the smell of these chemicals remains in the class even on the next day. Chemical residues often induce negative reactions in very sensitive people. Children place their hands on chairs and tables and end up inhaling the smell. They may even wind up in the child's mouth thus making him sensitive. The chemicals affect the brain functioning and in turn behavior. It has been observed that after parents and teachers wipe the students' desks with water or a natural cleaning solution prior to class each morning, they have reported rather remarkable improvements in the behavior of autistic children.

One can check if there are any early intervention programs that are available in the locality. The school district authorities can be contacted for evaluation of the child and thus the child can be enrolled for any special pre school program on the advice of a specialist. Make can also make a special request to the local school authorities and check whether they have any special programs for autistic children. The child needs to qualify for the special program and one should make sure that the school has set up an individual Education Plan for the child. This document is a very serious document that ensures that the child gets the special service and education needs. The free and appropriate education that is given to the child is called FAPE.

One can refer to some good parenting theory books that will help in the treatment of autistic children. There are many guides that are available and one may take recourse to them for help.

Autistic patients both young and old need constant care and attention. Autistic adults can be classified into two categories and they are High Functioning Autistics and Low Functioning Autistics (LFA). There are numerous health care professionals and organizations that can offer valuable advice on how to deal with these patients.

The high functioning autistic adults are very successful and they live relatively normal lives. They can work, care and support themselves and live independently with a family of their own. To lead a normal life the HFA adult must have had a proper education while growing up and if he has been effectively taught he can understand social behavior and responses. By the time the child reaches adulthood then he can adjust and contribute to society. Some high functioning autistics may still face or have to struggle with social interaction. There are organizations which health care providers that can help them and they can be consulted for support and guidance. The Low Functioning Autistics (LFA) need constant care and attention like autistic children. They too should be taken to health care specialists for guidance and proper progress evaluation.

There are a number of approaches that are used in the treatment and therapy of autistic patients. Some of the most popular ones are the structured and language therapy, social skills therapy and occupational therapy. Health care professionals' resorts to these natural therapy tools to treat patients and in the event of extreme cases they resort to medications. The healthcare professionals keep a daily track of neuropsychological reports to monitor progress and developments.

Autism is not a disorder to be dreaded and with professional guidance and personal evaluation a patient can lead a normal life. With family love and support an autistic patient can be successfully treated. Autism is not a disease it is a disorder that requires compassion, constant care and a supportive and understanding attitude towards the patient. There are many organizations that extend support and generate awareness on autism. Families of autistic patients can take recourse to these organizations and get invaluable advice and support for dealing with autistic patients and their well-being. Both parents and professionals can benefit from these programs and hence make autistic patients live a more better and fulfilled life.

REVIEW QUESTIONS FOR THE BONUS READING SECTION

1. The ideal caregiver is someone who knows his/her responsibilities, maintain punctuality very open to suggestions and takes pride in his/her job

   A. True

   B. False

   C. Neither

2. The responsibilities of the caregiver include all of the following except

   A. Routine personal care hygiene assistance

   B. Prescribing medications

   C. Rides to doctor appointments and errands

3. _____ is define as skillfulness by virtue a possessing special knowledge

   A. Limitations

   B. Identification

   C. Professionalism

4. A caregiver should always wear tight fitting jeans or pants to work

   A. True

   B. False

   C. Neither

5. Should you maintain personal hygiene as a caregiver

   A. Sometimes

   B. Always

   C. Never

6. _____ means the quality or habit of adhering to an appointed time

   A. Responsibility

   B. Professional

   C. Punctuality

7. If you find your patient slump all of a sudden while eating at the dining table what should you do?

   A. Call 911, start CPR, call your agency

   B. Run

C. Just ignore your patient because you are just there to make money

8. An ideal caregiver does not adjust to the needs of the patient

    A. True

    B. False

    C. Neither

9. Some problems that could occur when caregivers put themselves last include all of the following except

    A. Meeting their own needs

    B. They become ill and hate their job

    C. They do not deliver appropriate care to their patient

10. The United States made three 12 hour shifts full time to burn out caregivers

    A. True

    B. False

    C. Neither

11. If you want to be an ideal care giver then you need to stay in good health

    A. True

    B. False

    C. Neither

12. As a caregiver you should keep your own self updates about the disability or disease of the patient

    A. True

    B. False

    C. Neither

13. Bad communication is believed to be the most viable quality of a caregiver

    A. True

    B. False

    C. Neither

14. The 3 areas involve in keeping yourself safe as a caregiver involve all of the following except

    A. The five senses

    B. Information, sexual behaviors

C. Interrogating the patient

15. Some of the signs of frustration are

    A. Feeling happy

    B. Singing all the time

    C. Headache, knot in throat, desire to strike out

16. Calming down is necessary when there are any tensed situations involving the patient

    A. True

    B. False

    C. Neither

17. Any uncontrollable situations should be dealt with right away

    A. True

    B. False

    C. Neither

18. Some common ways of decreasing your stress involves all of the following except

    A. Meeting physical needs

    B. Praise your self

C. Going on a romantic date with your patient

19. Bad communication with the patient or to someone related with the patient is not important

    A. True

    B. False

    C. Neither

20. _____ communication is a form of expressing that is ineffective and maladaptive

    A. Passive communication

    B. Aggressive communication

    C. Good communication

21. The most effective and healthiest form of communication is the _____ style

    A. Aggressive

    B. Passive

    C. Assertive

22. Assertive style of communication is the style people use most

    A. True

B. False

C. Neither

23. There are _____ communication technique which can help get your message across towards the patient

A. 3

B. 5

C. 7

24. The first and foremost thing is to put our selves in their shoes

A. True

B. False

C. Neither

25. Listening carefully and respectfully to the values and beliefs of the patients and respecting them in your day to day activity is what is referred to as

A. Cultural activity

B. Assessment sensitivity

C. Cultural sensitivity

26. _____ is referred to as the way of life of the people

    A. Norms

    B. Culture

    C. Beliefs

27. Advantages of cultural sensitivity involves all of the following except

    A. Avoidance of conflicts

    B. A stronger connection with the client and the family members

    C. Respecting your own feelings, desires and needs

28. Communication is not the best way to negotiate with any differences arising out of cultural sensitivity

    A. True

    B. False

    C. Neither

29. Escorting a patient should not be confused with accompanying a patient to a destination

    A. True

B. False

C. Neither

30. A person who is escorting and transporting a patient should not be aware of the medical history and the clinical condition of the patient

   A. True

   B. False

   C. Neither

31. Some of the probable reasons of a fire breakout are smoking, cooking and a couple of other fire hazards

   A. True

   B. False

   C. Neither

32. The battery of the alarms needs to be charged at least _____ in a year

   A. Twice

   B. Checked

   C. Once

33. Politeness and simplicity is the only manners needed in conducting proper phone etiquette

    A. True

    B. False

    C. Neither

34. With aging the risk for falling increases because their senses dim and nervous systems tends to deteriorate

    A. True

    B. False

    C. Neither

35. It is true that most of the falls lead to minor injuries, but at the same time nearly _____ to _____ percent lead to fractures as well as other serious injuries

    A. Ten, sixty

    B. Ten, fifty

    C. Ten, seventy

36. Injuries that can result out of falls are broken bones, head injuries and even accidents that harm the interior body parts

    A. True

    B. False

    C. Neither

37. _____ is a common form of dementia in which a person faces problem with their memory or thought process

    A. Lupus

    B. COPD

    C. Alzheimer's

38. The symptoms of Alzheimer's are divided in two categories: _____ stage and _____ stage

    A. Late, noon

    B. Early, late

    C. Early, evening

39. The emotional support needs to come from the side of the caregiver and this can create a sense of wellbeing in the patient

   A. True

   B. False

   C. Neither

40. The early stage of Alzheimer attacks the patient so badly that they are not even in a position to communicate properly and they are completely dependent on the caregiver

   A. True

   B. False

   C. Neither

41. Memory loss in the Alzheimer's disease doesn't mean that the patient loses their feelings

   A. True

   B. False

   C. Neither

42. The last stage of Alzheimer's completely cripples a person both mentally as well as physically

   A. True

   B. False

   C. Neither

43. _____ is a brain disorder that deals with an abnormal self-absorption with oneself

   A. Alzheimer's

   B. Mad cow

   C. Autism

44. Autistic children tend to play repetitive games with toys for example lining up of objects and the turning on and off of light switches despite repeated scolding

   A. True

   B. False

   C. Neither

45. Some physical characteristic of autism may include

   A. They are neat and well behave

B. They communicate with adults only

C. The skin is pale, face has low muscle tone

46. There is laboratory tests to confirm autism

    A. True

    B. False

    C. Neither

47. The autistic patient may have fixations like making

    repeated noises, staring at turning wheels etc.

    A. True

    B. False

    C. Neither

48. Autistic individuals often have good auditory

    processing skills

    A. True

    B. False

    C. Neither

49. The high functioning autistic adults are very

    successful and they live relatively normal lives

    A. True

B. False

C. Neither

50. The _____ adult autistics need constant care
and attention like autistic children

A. Low functioning

B. High function

C. Normal functioning

HOME HEALTH AIDES SAMPLE QUESTIONS
ANSWERS

1) A
2) D
3) A
4) D
5) C
6) D
7) B
8) B
9) B
10) C
11) A
12) B
13) C

14) D

15) D

16) B

17) D

18) B

19) A

20) B

21) C

22) D

23) A

24) C

25) D

26) B

27) A

28) D

29) C

30) B

31) C

32) A

33) A

34) A

35) D

36) C

37) D

38) C

39) C

40) D

41) A

42) C

43) D

44) C

45) D

46) C

47) B

48) A

49) D

50) D

51) D

52) B

53) C

54) A

55) B

56) C

57) D

58) True

59) A

60) B

61) D

62) B

63) A

64) A

65) A

66) B

67) D

68) B

69) A

70) D

71) D

72) A

73) D

74) B

75) B

76) A

77) C

78) C

79) D

80) A

81) A

82) D

83) D

84) B

85) D

86) C

87) A

88) A

89) B

90) D

91) D

92) C

93) A

94) D

95) D

96) B

97) C

98) D
99) A
100) A

ANSWERS FOR THE BONUS READING FOR HOME CAREGIVERS

1. A
2. B
3. C
4. B
5. B
6. C
7. A
8. B
9. A
10. B
11. A
12. A
13. B
14. C
15. C
16. A
17. B
18. C
19. B
20. A

21. C
22. B
23. B
24. A
25. C
26. B
27. C
28. B
29. A
30. B
31. A
32. C
33. B
34. A
35. B
36. A
37. C
38. B
39. A
40. B
41. A
42. A
43. C
44. A
45. C
46. B
47. A
48. B
49. A
50. A

THER TITLES FROM THE SAME AUTHOR:

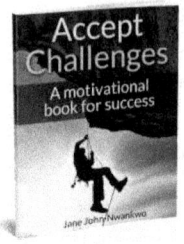
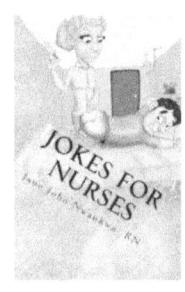
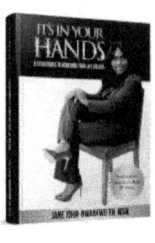

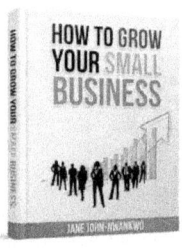
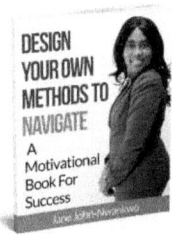
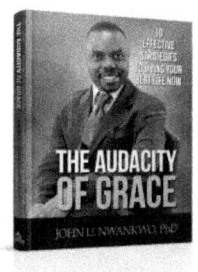

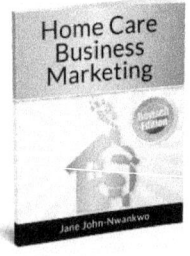
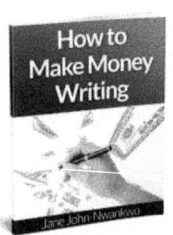
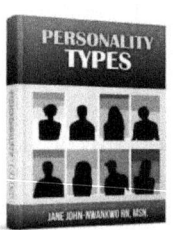

www.djngbooks.org

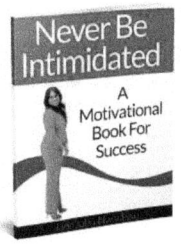

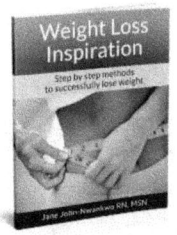

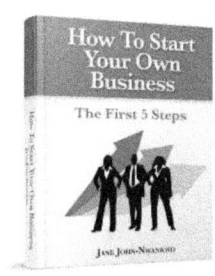

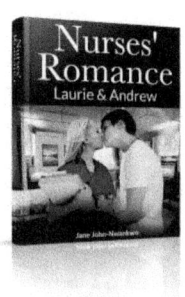

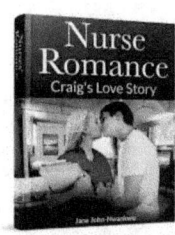

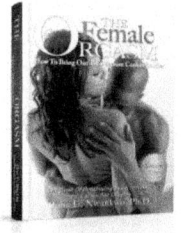

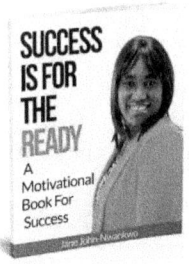

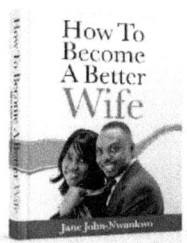

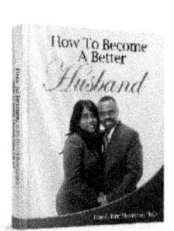

www.janejohn-nwankwo.com

ABOUT THE AUTHOR

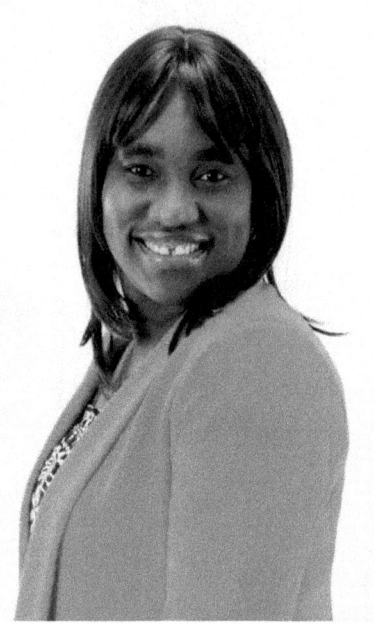

Jane John-Nwankwo CPT, RN, MSN, PHN is a motivational speaker and published author of more than 50 books which include textbooks for healthcare training, fiction for entertainment, and motivational books.
Simply search
"Books by Jane John-Nwankwo"
On Amazon.com

Visit her website:
www.janejohn-nwankwo.com

Book Jane John-Nwankwo as your motivational speaker now at www.JaneJohn-Nwankwo.com

With more than 10 years as a professional speaker, Jane John-Nwankwo can hold any audience sitting straight on their chairs for any length of time! She is a seminar leader and a published author of more than 50 books including textbooks for healthcare training, fiction for entertainment, books for new entrepreneurs and motivational and inspirational books like the "It's in your hands" series.

She earned her Masters of Science in Nursing from University of Phoenix, and is currently pursuing a PhD in Nursing Science. Her speaking interests include: Motivational speeches for new business owners, Motivational speeches for any category of people, Employee seminars, Students' Empowerment, Healthcare topics, Topics related to women and any Christian topic. Book a speaking appointment today Wow! your audience. Electrify your seminar!!

www.janejohn-nwankwo.com

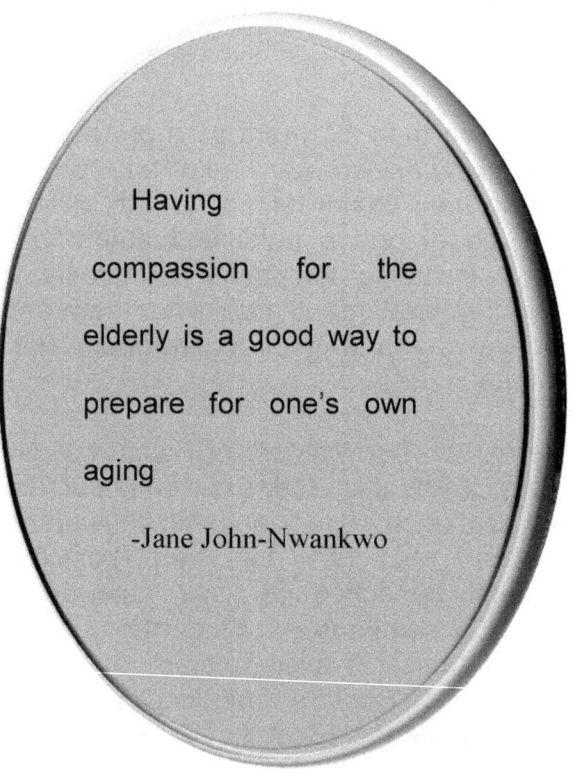

Having

compassion for the

elderly is a good way to

prepare for one's own

aging

-Jane John-Nwankwo